ESSENTIAL OILS HAVE SUPER POWERS®

From Solving Everyday Wellness Problems with Aromatherapy to Taking on "Superbugs"

By Kathy Heshelow
Sublime Beauty Naturals® and Zen Box
Member, NAHA

Essential Oils Have Super Powers®; From Solving Everyday Problems with Aromatherapy to Taking on "Superbugs". 2nd edition.

ISBN 978-1-4951-9496-2 (book) - ISBN 978-0-692-65198-8 (ebook)

Published by Sublime Beauty Naturals®
11125 Park Blvd, Suite 104-103, Seminole FL 33772
ISBN 978-1-4951-9496-2 (book) - ISBN 978-0-692-65198-8 (ebook)

Heshelow portrait by Heidi Haponowitz Photography

Printed in the United States

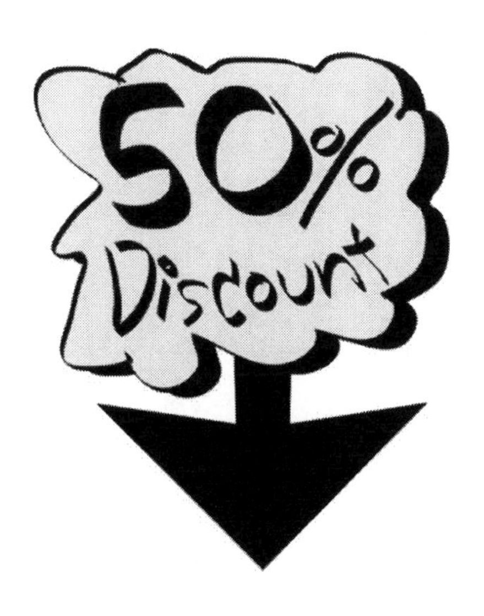
50%
Discount

Disclaimer

This book and information is for reference and education, and represents my views and research, including the research, publications and clinical tests of others. Essential oils and aromatherapy, for me, support what the body needs and requires to thrive, and they work at the holistic level of mind-body-spirit.

I fully stand behind the natural wellness properties of essential oils, using them in my daily life. However, the statements in this book are not intended as a substitute for professional healthcare nor meant to diagnose, cure or prevent medical conditions or serious disease.

Every illness or injury requires supervision by a medical doctor, integrative doctor and/or an alternative medicine practitioner such as a certified holistic doctor or certified aromatherapist practitioner.

Preface

Welcome to the updated 2nd edition of this book, including the cover. There are not many changes – mostly in the antibiotic-resistant bacteria chapter and new research added in Chapter 3!

Essential oils are enchanting yet powerful – and so much fun to use and learn about. The book was a joy to initially write in early 2016, and it has been fun revisiting it this year. I hope you enjoy it!

I feel so strongly about the valuable powers of essential oils that I trademarked the title of the book and the phrase: Essential Oils have Super Powers®! Some might be curious about this phrase, others might think it is hyperbole, or roll their eyes. Those in the know will shake their head in agreement right away. In any case, I explain my reasoning throughout the book, and my reasoning will become quite clear.

Let me say this right away: essential oils do not "cure" every malady under the sun (as some websites or companies would have you believe), but they do have strong natural powers that benefit us in so many fabulous ways; they can indeed help or even speed the healing process and improve specific conditions; and they add joy to our daily lives in a natural way, as you will learn in this book.

I have been using essential oils for a long time. I lived in Paris, France for 16 years, where essential oils are more commonly used and understood in everyday life, and accepted by the medical world. (And oh, those summer trips to the south of France where fields of lavender and other fragrant plants thrived!) You can find essential oils and products in the local pharmacies, and doctors may suggest them for treatment in France. Hospitals or clinics may diffuse certain oils because they kill microbes. (You will learn in this book why France and Europe in general are more advanced in this regard and why the approach is different than in the U.S.)

My first two early essential oil (EO) loves years ago were Eucalyptus and Geranium. Eucalyptus helped (and still does today) keep my sinuses clear and congestion down. Geranium is a wonderful essential oil for balance and uplift of spirit, and I often diffuse it in my office (along with my current favorite Frankincense and daily topical application of Zen Immune Boost Blend.) My mom had pots of geranium flowers in my bedroom windowsill, shared with my sister when I was growing up. I still remember awaking to the wonderful aroma, seeing the beautiful flowers, and associate it with good thoughts.

While essential oils - or at least aromatic plants - have been in use for thousands of years (read the intriguing history section that includes the caves of Lascaux in France, ancient Egypt, Persia, China, ancient Greece and Rome, Ayurvedic India, and the Renaissance), the more "modern" use really started in France thanks to René-Maurice Gattefossé, considered the father of aromatherapy. Ah, France once again!

For my part, I love that essential oils are a blend of old and new approaches to wellness, and that they are entirely natural and of the earth, extracted from plants. They share their natural powers with us (*did you know that plant and human DNA is extremely similar?*), working with the mind, body and spirit to improve wellness - alone or in concert with the traditional medical modalities. The traditional U.S. medical world typically overlooks mind and spirit when treating a condition... and they often work only to deal with symptoms of the body rather than the holistic view or the source of the problem, though this is starting to change.

Essential oils have so many different benefits and can be a complementary force for wellness. You will be amazed when you read about some of the ways they can help you and your family, and some of the clinical research being done today.

Essential oils? They awaken our senses; they can help with such conditions as depression, memory loss, sleeplessness, pain, focus, memory and anxiety. They can help improve our immune system. They can help create a tranquil environment, or one with energy. They can help with inflammation or specific injury healing (such as cuts, burns and bites). They can kill bacteria and microbes,

cleanse our homes naturally, and so much more. This is why, to me, they have super powers!

Because I love these precious oils and use them frequently, I decided to take it to a more formal level with an intense certification training (ACP certification, 235 hours, internationally recognized, currently studying at Aromahead Institute headed by Andrea Butje).

For my business, I offer the best therapeutic-grade essential oils I can find (with GC/MS testing available to any buyer) through my company Sublime Beauty Naturals®. My mission has been to offer education and safety tips for those entering the market!

The motto of Sublime Beauty Naturals®:

MAKE HEALTHY CHOICES, RESPECT YOUR BODY, LOVE NATURE

And that motto sums up my view on essential oils! Using them can be a meaningful choice for your wellness and shows respect for your body as well as the power of nature. Essential oils enhance and support what the body needs to thrive, as naturally as possible, with as little side effects as possible, and complementing wellness.

Finally, I am so proud to be a contributing producer on the documentary film in progress, "Uncommon Scents". It's all about Aromatherapy and essential oils, being made by Angela Jensen Ehmke and Kristina Bauer (Executive Producers). Ehmke directs and Bauer writes, with eminent figures like Robert Tisserand in the film. I believe this documentary will help improve the knowledge, interest, education and understanding of essential oils, which is long overdue! The movie is anticipated in 2017-2018.

I hope you enjoy this book!

WHAT IS MY WISH? If you are not already enchanted by the super powers of Essential Oils, you may become so!

~ Kathy Heshelow
www.kathyheshelow.com | www.BooksByHeshelow.com

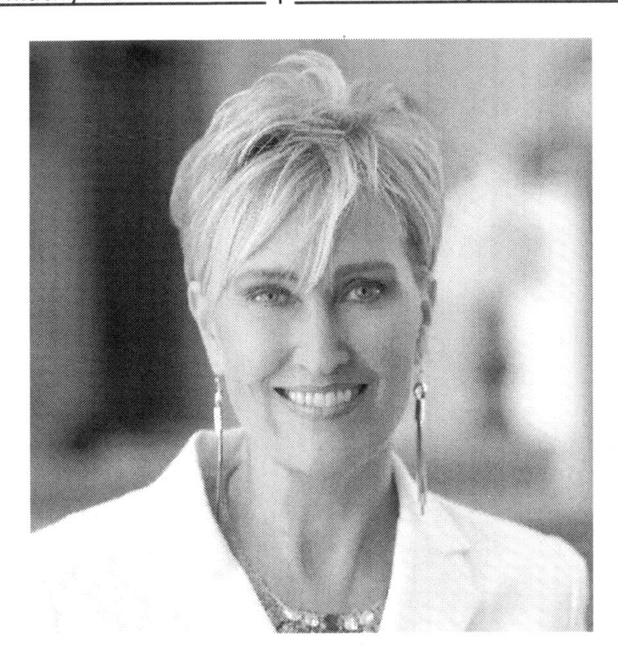

Acknowledgements

There are so many legends and pioneers in the field of aromatherapy and essential oil work, and as I have studied and absorbed the information, I try to bring them into this book, credit their work and share what is important.

I give special recognition to many, and thanks for their studies, research and education: Robert Tisserand, Dr. Kurt Schaubelt, Dr. David Crow, Dr. Rodney Young, Dr. Joshua Plant, Dr. Joie Powers, Dr. Scott A Johnson, Dr. Joshua Plant, Dr. Mercola, Sayer Ji of GreenMedInfo, Dr. Axe, Darren Moore, Ashley Rivers, Dr. Rory Stern, Jamie Garvey at Boswellness, Aromatherapy Thymes magazine, Cari Romm and Tori Rodrigues of The Atlantic, and Dana Ullman of the Huffington Post, and NAHA (the National Association of Holistic Aromatherapy); and Andrea Butje and her team at Aromahead Institute. From the past, influences include: Rene-Maurice Gattefossé, Dr. Jean Valnet, Marguerite Maury, and Henri Viaud. Thanks to my early ZEN BOX family as well!

And of course, I thank my great husband, Harlan, who is always supportive!

TABLE OF CONTENTS

PREFACE 5

ACKNOWLEDGEMENTS 10

TABLE OF CONTENTS 11

INTRODUCTION 13

SAFETY FIRST 16

CHAPTER 1 23

WHAT ARE THESE THINGS CALLED ESSENTIAL OILS – AND WHY DO THEY HAVE SUPER POWERS? 23

CHAPTER 2 55

FASCINATING HISTORY: AROMATIC PLANTS TO ESSENTIAL OILS 55

CHAPTER 3 102

THE WOW FACTOR: CLINICAL RESEARCH & STUDIES OF ESSENTIAL OILS 102

CHAPTER 4 166

THE CRISIS OF "SUPERBUGS", ANTIBIOTICS AND ESSENTIAL OILS 166

CHAPTER 5 207

DIFFERENT APPROACHES TO ESSENTIAL OILS AROUND THE WORLD 207

CHAPTER 6 232

MIND – BODY – SPIRIT AND AROMATHERAPY 232

CHAPTER 7 254

MAGIC OF EXTRACTION... AND "CONSTITUENTS" THAT DEFINE THEIR POWER 254

CHAPTER 8 263

MY TOP 15 ESSENTIAL OILS, BENEFITS AND PROPERTIES.............. 263

CHAPTER 9.. 302

SOME SIMPLE & HELPFUL BLENDING RECIPES + TYPICAL DILUTIONS
.... 302

CHAPTER 10.. 319

CARING FOR YOUR ESSENTIAL OILS.. 319

REFERENCES.. 322

BIBLIOGRAPHY.. 340

ABOUT THE AUTHOR.. 343

INTRODUCTION

"Health is a state of body. Wellness is a state of being." ~J. Stanford

"The intimate connection of essential oils to the evolution of enzymes in our bodies is but one factor that demonstrates how essential oils have naturally, from time immemorial, interfaced with humans." ~ Dr. Schnaubelt

If you have picked up this book, you might be new to essential oils and want to learn what they are all about. But you could just as well be an expert quite familiar with this world, and want to see what I have to say! The book is meant to serve both audiences.

What the book is not? It is not a technical guide, nor one that goes deep into the chemical components, constituents or molecular science. Though I share some good basic recipes for common ailments, it does not contain endless recipes for all ailments (see my book USE THIS FOR THAT! for this angle!), nor does it include how to make skincare creams, soaps, candles and such. There are many such guides available online and in books.

I have tried to share some different information not found in many books currently available – more details than typically found on the fascinating history of essential oils and aromatic plants (Chapter 2), current and recent research work in such areas as superbugs and the antibiotic crisis that affect us all – and the role essential oils may play (will play, in my opinion – Chapters 3 and 4). This includes the antibiotic-resistant bacterial issues with our food supply. I have tried to aggregate a selection of research references in Chapter 3 – not only for those who want to investigate further, but to show just a glimpse of the amount and the kinds of research going on.

I take a look at why there are differences in the way essential oils are viewed, accepted, applied and used in different countries (Chapter 5); and more on the mind-body-spirit connection (Chapter 6) along with new related areas of science and how emotion actually affects genes and longevity. I don't overlook distillation methods and constituents of essential oils that are pertinent (Chapter 7).

There are many encyclopedias of essential oils, and books devoted to profiling them in depth, so I have kept this section to a minimum. I include interesting profiles on my personal choice of top 15 essential oils (Chapter 8), plus the most basic and useful of my favorite recipes for common issues you encounter in your life (Chapter 9).

Don't forget - there are hundreds of essential oils! I concentrate on the ones that are extremely helpful and more commonly found in the U.S. – and if you are new to essential oils, ones you may want to start with. I finish with the easy steps of caring for your essential oils (Chapter 10).

Let's start with Safety First!

~ Kathy Heshelow

SAFETY FIRST

Before we get into all of the information, history and power of essential oils, I wanted to point out safety precautions first. Do take a moment to go over the list if you are going to use or experiment with essential oils. Don't overlook this!

Essential oils are pure and natural plant-based essences and as such are generally considered to be relatively safe. It is very hard to overdose on them when used topically or by inhaling, and most essential oils do not cause side effects like some traditional medicines can.

HOWEVER, you should be very aware of the following *(and understand this may not be a complete safety reference.)* If you have any questions, please reach out, consult your physician if you have any physical ailment or are in traditional treatment with medication(s), or consult your certified aromatherapist, integrative or holistic doctor.

✓ A good rule of thumb is to not use a pure single essential oil undiluted directly on skin, also called using it "neat", before doing a test-patch. Many are too concentrated and could irritate the skin. Exceptions for using essential oils neat may be made for some like lavender, helichrysum, frankincense, and rose geranium. In the U.S., it is typical to find warnings against using all essential oils undiluted, but they are regularly used so in some countries and can be quite helpful in some situations (such as lavender or rose geranium on a burn or cut.)

- ✓ We like to recommend a small skin patch test prior to <u>every first-time</u> use of an essential oil or blend, just to be safe. If any reaction occurs, use an oil or milk to wipe it off (an oil will help dilute the essential oils and sooth the skin.) You can then use plentiful soap and water on the patch area. (Reactions are not common.)

- ✓ Keep essential oils away from your eyes! In the event of eye Injury from an EO, irrigate eye with a sterile saline solution for 15 minutes. Immediately consult a physician if pain persists after the eye wash.

- ✓ In general, we DO NOT recommend that essential oils be ingested. Some oils could be toxic if ingested even in small amounts, and poisoning of children has occurred. Essential oils are highly concentrated and strong – and if we test them on our skin undiluted, you would want to be careful to expose your mouth, esophagus, intestines, mucus membranes and body organs. There are instances when a licensed medical practitioner or certified aromatherapist may treat with internal use (typically in capsules or a few drops in a liquid), but this is more common in Europe and only with specific EOs and specific ailments. While it may be a practice that exists, it's best not to experiment. (I write more about this in Chapter 1.)

- ✓ Keep essential oils in a locked cabinet, away from small children. Children (especially toddlers) can be fascinated with the look and smell of essential oils. If accidental ingestion occurs contact poison control immediately.

- ✓ Babies, pets and elderly persons require lower doses of essential oils, half that recommended for a healthy adult (or even less, depending on the essential oil). Peppermint and eucalyptus have been known to cause respiratory problems with young babies or the elderly. Lavender and neroli, despite their gentle nature, can be tolerated only in very small amounts (1 drop in bath water and 1/2 drop per ounce of carrier oil.) We highlight dilution and dosage recommendations in Chapter 9.

- ✓ Essential Oils are highly flammable; use extreme care around fire.

- ✓ Cancer patients may use mild dilutions of bergamot, chamomile, lavender, ginger and frankincense; however, fennel and aniseed in particular should be avoided.

- ✓ Persons undergoing chemotherapy should avoid using essential oils <u>during</u> chemo unless prescribed by a licensed or certified practitioner. (Peppermint may be an exception, as it could help with nausea.) Tisserand and Young have written about essential oils during chemotherapy or radiation in their book "Essential Oil Safety: A Guide for Healthcare Professionals". (1). There is some question as to whether antioxidant essential oils that protect normal cells could also protect cancerous cells that the treatment is meant to eliminate.

✓ All oils containing eugenol (Clove), thymol (Thyme) and carvacrol (Oregano) should be avoided by people taking anticoagulant medication, those with clotting or bleeding disorders, major surgery, childbirth, peptic ulcer or hemophilia. These components "thin" the blood and could cause excessive bleeding.

✓ Asthma and epilepsy patients should avoid fennel, hyssop and rosemary – and in my opinion, asthma sufferers should proceed with caution in general when introducing new essential oils into their environment or topically on the body. Some can and will be helpful indeed, but asthma sufferers are more sensitive and susceptible.

- ✓ High blood pressure patients should avoid black pepper, clove, hyssop, peppermint, rosemary, sage and thyme essential oils.

- ✓ Low blood pressure patients should avoid excessive use of lavender oil.

- ✓ Diabetics should not use angelica.

- ✓ Those who suffer from hypoglycemia should stay away from geranium (rose geranium). Sufferers of kidney problems should be cautious if they use juniper, sandalwood, or coriander.

- ✓ Clary Sage should not be used while drinking as it will intensify the effects of the alcohol, causing it to act like a narcotic.

- ✓ Chamomile and Marjoram should not be used while driving because they cause drowsiness, and as noted above, be careful of too much Lavender when driving.

- ✓ Methyl salicylate is the active ingredient in aspirin as well as sweet birch and wintergreen essential oil. If you use aspirin for medicinal purposes you should avoid sweet birch or wintergreen due to the risk of overdose. It should also be kept away from children as it smells sweet and is equally dangerous to them.

- ✓ Pregnant women should avoid essential oils before the 18th week of pregnancy, especially in cases of prior miscarriage. In the second trimester, essential oils may possible be used in low doses ONLY if formulated by a professional aromatherapist or health care provider. To be safe, wait until the third trimester, until after birth, or consult a doctor.

- ✓ Essential Oils to avoid in general: Mugwart, Pennyroyal, Rue and Sage.

OK, let's get to the fun!

CHAPTER 1

WHAT ARE THESE THINGS CALLED ESSENTIAL OILS – AND WHY DO THEY HAVE SUPER POWERS?

Aromatherapy is not a luxury. It is an inexpensive way to maintain health and to treat many diseases naturally.
~ Kurt Schnaubelt, Ph.D.

Only the educated are free.
~Epictetus (55-135 A.D.)

Essential oils, pure and simple, are the concentrated aromatic essences extracted from certain plants. Essential oils are sometimes called the "life force" or "soul" of a plant.

The word "oil" itself is a bit of a misnomer, as essential oils don't have the fatty acid component necessary for a true oil. These precious liquids are commonly more thin and watery than oily; they are powerful substances considered to be the "plant's physician". Highly concentrated and volatile (meaning they evaporate quickly), essential oils typically contain valuable organic components.

Each essential oil will contain many different chemical compounds and constituents, each of which exhibits a specific therapeutic property. In general, essential oils can be subdivided into two distinct groups of chemical constituents; the hydrocarbons which are made up almost exclusively of terpenes (monoterpenes, sesquiterpenes, and diterpenes), and the oxygenated compounds which are mainly esters, aldehydes, ketones, alcohols, phenols, and oxides. (You'll learn details about compounds and constituents, and what they can do in Chapter 7.)

What gives an essential oil its special powers and uniqueness is not just one or two of its constituents but the entire complexity and makeup.

Essential oils are energetic, dynamic and unique.

Essential oils are used in aromatherapy (inhaled or

used topically) for physical and emotional balance and wellness. They are also found in some skincare products, cleaning products, candles and soaps. Some are used in perfumes (though many in perfumes are synthetic or "watered down", not true essential oils). In this book, I am for the most part writing about pure therapeutic essential oils extracted from plants and used singly or in blends for aromatherapy or therapeutic use.

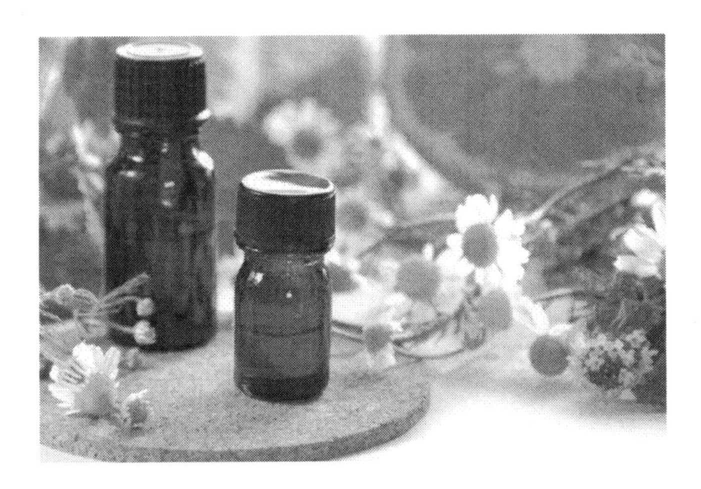

WHY DO ESSENTIAL OILS HAVE SUPER POWERS? HERE IS MY SHORT SUMMARY:

Essential Oils are complex precious oils that give us aid to heal; the power to kill microbes; the power of protection; and the power of joy of scent.

Different Essential Oils can bring vitality or relaxation;
They can support the immune system or improve memory;
They can help reduce stress or anxiety;
They can help improve the ability to sleep or reduce congestion;
They can help reduce depression or burn-out;
They reduce or kill viruses or bacteria in the air;
They can help reduce headaches;
They help with inflammation and wound-healing;
They can help improve alertness and concentration;
They can help ease the pain or nausea, indigestion or cramps;
They are shown to assist with a number of conditions, such as ADHD and PTSD as well as helping with Alzheimer's and Dementia patients in clinical tests; and MUCH MUCH more.

Essential Oils can be used for preventative care (like keeping your immune system strong) as well as for active care (like reducing an anxiety attack or healing a burn).

Each oil holds many powers and can adapt to what the body needs. They are intelligent and versatile.

Essential Oils do all this with the power of nature. Imagine a plant, in one place without the ability to run away or hide from predators or pathogens, rooted in place. They must produce their own defenses, which is what essential oils are and what they do. They help the plant to repel or attract, they protect against pathogens, etc.

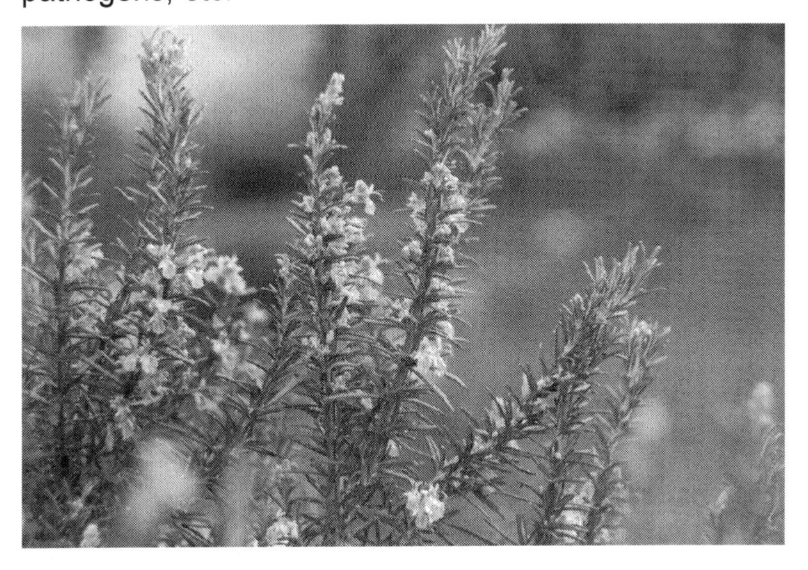

And plant DNA is very close to our DNA. This is what makes them so beneficial to us – the natural protective powers against various pathogens - with certain metabolite powers to improve and strengthen wellness. Essential oils accomplish this for the most part without side effects that typical pharmaceuticals may have (many pharmaceuticals in fact try to copy plants and their powers.) Drugs, especially antibiotics), and toxins may kill good flora in the gut or body thereby lowering our level of health, or create unwanted side effects. Essential oils do not create these side effects or toxins. And this is one reason why I have assigned them the "super power" status!

Psssst - while most Essential Oils smell pleasant, this is just a happy coincidence and an added joy to their real benefits.

Essential Oils can make our everyday life healthier, happier or more balanced. They can be used to substitute out household cleaners, bug killers, gardening chemicals, mold removers and toxic products found in many everyday items. Almost any common condition you may suffer could be addressed with an essential oil for help. And they have a role to play in combating antibiotic-resistant bacteria and microbes, too. I devote a full chapter to this subject.

TOXINS ABOUND

We are assaulted by hundreds of toxins every single day, in our water, food and household products, cleaners and personal care items (preservatives, pesticides, dyes, additives, hormones). Many antibiotics can cause as much harm as good, and poor use of them has enabled “superbugs”. Our bodies take in these toxins and then the lymphatic system works to get them out – and we are often just overloaded. These toxins can create a range of problems from allergies and low energy to serious diseases.

Did you know that many chemicals banned in Europe and elsewhere are commonly found in U.S. products? (This includes antibiotics given to chickens and cows.) Even when you think you are using or eating “safe” products, this may be a fallacy. Toxins are simply everywhere. (1)

Trading out some of these toxic products we use in our homes with natural products relieves our body systems, improves wellness, helps the environment and supports organic farmers and manufacturers. This can help guard against disease weakening our systems, and help make our bodies stronger. The secondary metabolite powers of essential oils (that is, the essence that helps protect the plant survive against attacks or environmental hazards) transfers to us and helps us.

Many people who consistently use essential oils find that they get sick less often and their life is enhanced. One reason? Essential oils have the natural ability to eliminate toxins, bacteria and viruses.

Certain people and even whole towns involved in aromatic plants survived the medieval Plague, also known as The Black Death. About 40% of all Europeans died from it. Those who survived were often those who worked with essential oils, perfumes, plant essences and distilleries. The town of Bucklersbury in England was the center of the European Lavender trade and its residents for the most part stayed safe. A number of places in the south of France had a higher percentage of survivors (deep in the perfume and plant-based industries). And let's not forget the infamous "4 thieves of Marseilles", who immersed themselves in specific essential oil extracts and were able to steal and rob from Plague victims without getting sick.

ESSENTIAL OILS CAN DO THAT?

The most profound powers of essential oils, in my opinion, are due to antifungal, antibacterial, antiviral, anti-inflammatory and antispasmodic qualities. We highlight this in more detail in chapters 3 and 4, from clinical research which shows specific essential oils can kill all microbes in a room to an MRSA-infected patient in Australia who was facing amputation of a leg – but a treatment of essential oils was able to stop the antibiotic resistant disease, reverse it and heal the infection.

What else can essential oils do? Here are just a few examples of what some specific essential oils can do. You can see from these simple examples, one essential oil can do many things. In any case, they are versatile multi-taskers. For example:

- ✓ Lavender can work to calm, regularize and balance body and mind, help with sleep. It is a good essential oil to use on a burn or cut for strong healing powers.
- ✓ Eucalyptus can work to purify, clear, cool, and revitalize the body and mind. It is a good one to

use for colds and congestion, or sinus problems.

- ✓ Peppermint can invigorate, refresh, calm nausea, cool, and promote energy. There is an incredible list of what peppermint can do, including breaking sugar addiction and feel satiated. (2)
- ✓ Rosemary can warm, boost, heal and clarify body and mind, and help with memory.
- ✓ Sweet Orange can uplift, cheer and stimulate body and mind, and unclog oily skin pores.
- ✓ Geranium can stabilize, relax, help relieve grief and soothe body and mind. It helps bleeding to stop (or clot) and is good to use on a cut.
- ✓ Bergamot can normalize your mind, relax & build confidence and eases anxiety. It's a wonderful, lesser known citrus essential oil, great for cleansing and anti-bacterial use, too.
- ✓ Frankincense can encourage emotional healing, focus, support reflection and tranquility. It helps bring down inflammation well.

By inhaling directly, diffusing in a room, applying

topically (with a carrier oil) and/or massaging them in, your body takes in the goodness of the essential oil – whether inhaling in the pathway from the nose to the limbic system of the brain for action, or whether absorbing through the skin to the blood pathways for delivery.

Absorption and taking action in our body systems is actually strongest and fastest through inhalation, then second most effective is through topical use, says Dr. Joie Powers, PhD. (3)

HOW COME MY DOCTOR HASN'T TOLD ME ABOUT ESSENTIAL OILS?

Let's address this issue right away: if you are a newbie, you might think – how come my doctor hasn't suggested essential oils? Why haven't I heard about the ways essential oils can help from the hospital, clinic or my medical people? Are essential oils simply "hippy-new-age" things? Are they some kind of "snake oil"?

Unlike in other countries (and notably France and

Europe as well as some Asian countries), U.S. medical schools don't teach about essential oils or other "alternative" natural methods. So yes, if you go to a doctor, most of them are not talking about essential oils as they were simply not taught it in traditional education – although the growing trend of integrative care and doctors who are opening up to the natural healing power is increasing.

Major cancer centers are starting to use aromatherapy in the U.S. I see it more often in cancer centers and some major hospitals. My husband had knee replacement surgery, and the hospital offered aromatherapy for calming and reduction of pain, and there seems to be a growing awareness in the U.S. though it is still relatively unknown.

It seems that traditional medical establishments have mostly been influenced by research dollars, insurance and big pharmaceutical lobbies & companies (who have no interest in essential oils because they cannot trademark them.) So while you may not have heard of essential oils from your doctor and while you may in the future, it was worth mentioning this point here!

And you will discover that the powers of essential oils are real.

HOW DO ESSENTIAL OILS ENTER THE BODY AND WORK

There are three (3) ways for essential oils to enter your body and conduct their magic:

1) **Inhalation** through the nose to the brain and limbic system (and then dispersed in your body through the lungs and into the bloodstream)
2) **Absorption** through the skin when topically applied, to the bloodstream for delivery
3) **Internal ingestion** (not typically used in the U.S. and not recommended without professional supervision). Remember, this is called *aromatherapy.*

I, in fact, like the combination of inhalation and topical application for many of the oils and blends and this is a most effective approach. Inhalation is highly effective with a 70% average bioavailability. (Bioavailability is the proportion of a substance that enters in circulation when introduced into the body, giving ability to have an active effect.)

LIMBIC SYSTEM AND INHALATION

The role of inhalation of essential oils – it's all tied to our limbic system!

Did you know that your sense of smell is the ONLY of the five senses tied directly to the limbic system in your brain. This is the oldest area of the brain which deals with emotional and psychological responses.

The limbic system is like your control panel, for memory and formation of memories, emotion, sex drive, sleep cycles, thirst and physiological actions (like heart rate and breathing rate), time perception, instincts and motivation. The limbic system emerged and developed in the first mammals. (It is one step up from what is known as the reptilian brain.)

The limbic system consists of a complex set of structures that lies on both sides of the thalamus, just under the cerebrum. It includes the hypothalamus, the hippocampus, the amygdala, and several other sections.

The Limbic System

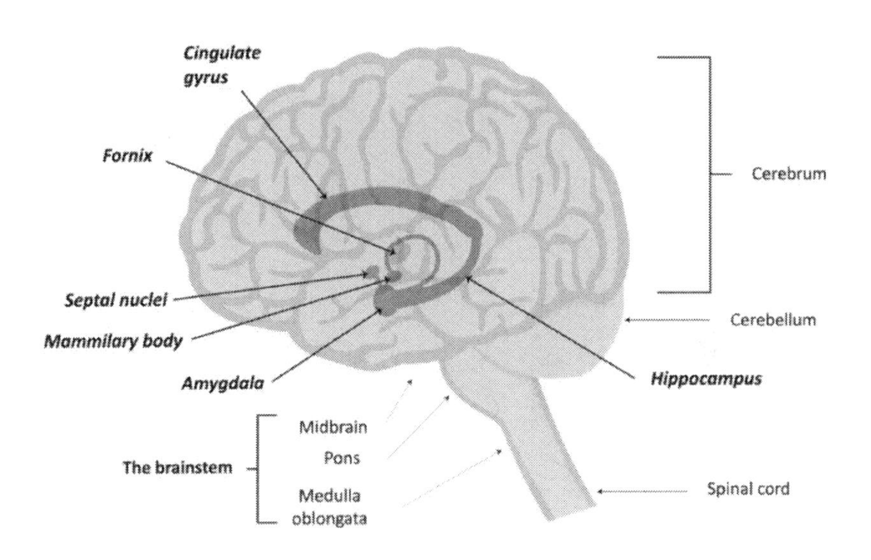

Some of the disorders associated with the limbic system are epilepsy and schizophrenia. Dysfunction or imbalance specifically within the amygdala often results in maladaptive social behavior, such as phobias, compulsions, paranoia and depression. (Some essential oils may be able to help balance these functions.)

When the nerve impulses are activated by scent, a reaction occurs – from calming to invigorating, from secretion of certain hormones or changing body systems (such as slowing the heart rate in an anxiety attack) - and the reaction occurs immediately.

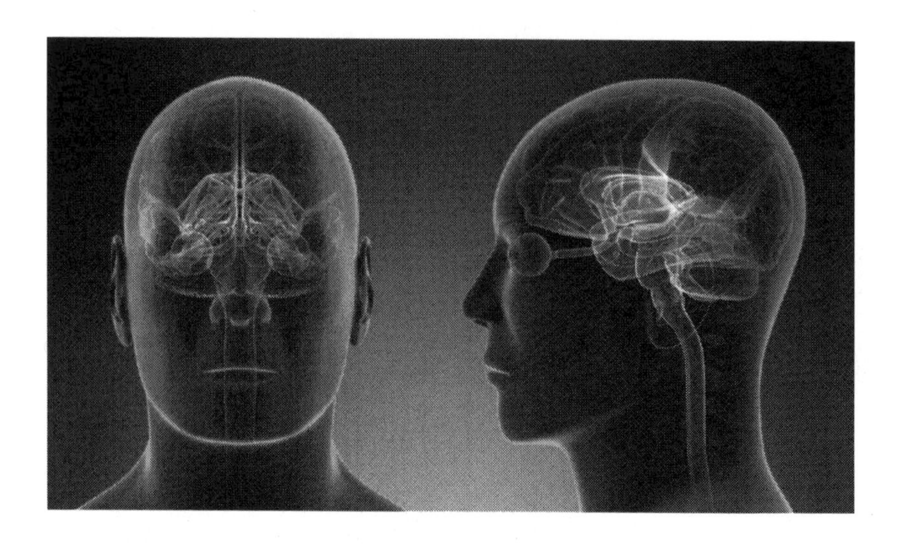

Think of how you react when you smell freshly cut grass, bread baking in the oven, a fresh Christmas tree, puppy breath or popcorn at the cinema. They are tied to your emotions and memory triggered in the brain and limbic system. When essential oils are inhaled, they travel from the nose directly to your brain control center! They promote the production and release of various neurotransmitters which impact your nervous system.

The other four senses — taste, sight, touch and hearing — are first routed through the thalamus before reaching designated areas of the brain. By the way, our sense of smell is estimated to be 10,000 times more acute than our other senses, and sensitive to millions of scents and aromas.

Note: Unlike many medicines or treatments for ailments, essential oils do not pass through the digestive system (unless ingested, of course).

Our sense of smell and the impact odors have on us (invoking emotions, actions or reactions) is a truly interesting area of study that is still not fully understood.

Depending on the chemical composition or constituents of an EO, every oil will excel in certain areas. The synergistic effects of the various constituents within an essential oil – all of the complex components – are what make it special and able to do many different things.

Some essential oils like rosemary bring down the cortisol level which can help calm us during anxiety (when cortisol levels shoot up), while others are stimulating like eucalyptus or lemon. Some are balancing like Roman chamomile or frankincense; eucalyptus may stimulate the immune system (specifically phagocytic response) (4).

As an essential oil or blend of essential oils travels through the nose to the limbic system, your brain receives signals for any needed physical, emotional and bodily reactions. Your body takes what is needed.

The synergistic effects of the various constituents within an essential oil – all of the complex components – are what make it special and able to do many different things.

Let's highlight a few examples or case studies:

In 1989, Dr. Joseph Ledoux at New York Medical University, discovered that the amygdala plays a role in storing and releasing emotional trauma. Essential oil therapy is now being used to help repair emotional trauma – from PTSD to rape victims. EOs have little side effects, compared to their pharmaceutical counterparts, which means more safety in healing trauma. From the studies of Dr. Hirsch, Dr. Ledoux and others, we can conclude that aromas may exert a profound effect in triggering a response or healing. (5a, 5b)

A study performed on students with ADHD ages 11-12 showed positive results when essential oils were used. The essential oils encouraged relaxation of the hyperactivity, and this helped improved concentration. Students stayed calmer longer, and recovered quickly from upsets. There were fewer disruptions to lessons.

In the same study, a blend of frankincense, Roman chamomile, lavender, bergamot, and mandarin was blended. This combination helped ease panic attacks and feelings of anxiety in an ADHD client. (6)

In studies performed in Vienna and Berlin Universities, researchers discovered that sesquiterpenes (a natural constituent found in essential oils such as vetiver, patchouli, cedarwood, sandalwood, and frankincense) can increase levels of oxygen in the brain by up to 28 percent. (7) This increase in oxygen could help an injured brain heal and resolve many issues, or possibly improve function of a healthy brain. It could improve learning and concentration while also helping to support immune and hormonal balances. An added bonus is that it could also lead to higher energy levels.

THE SECOND ROUTE OF DELIVERY: HOW DO ESSENTIAL OILS WORK IN TOPICAL APPLICATION?

Essential oils are made up of small molecules and when applied to the skin, are able to pass through the skin (strateum corneum including epidermis) down to the dermis and then into the bloodstream, to be delivered throughout the body. They are also able to cross the blood-brain barrier.

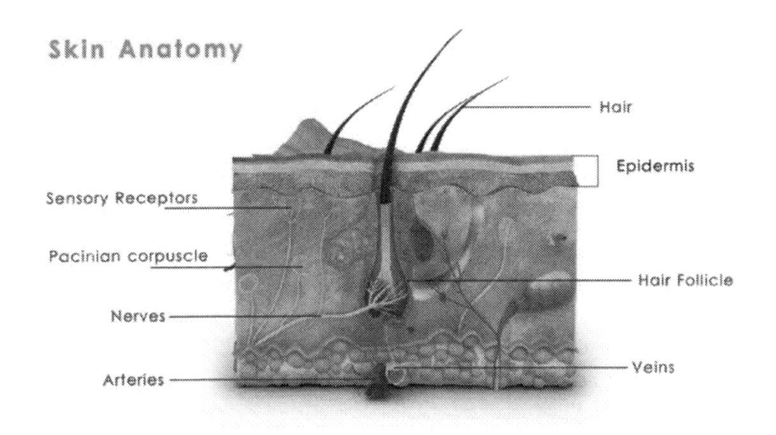

The carrier oil (that is, the oil used to dilute and blend the essential oils enabling topical use) and its viscosity will play a role in absorption. Some oils are quickly and easily absorbed (like jojoba or baobab) while others have thicker molecules and are slower to absorb (like avocado oil). Such factors as temperature, rate of blood circulation and other things also affect absorption.

In 1940 a researcher named Straehli did some fascinating tests on essential oils. He found that all the essential oils tested appeared in his subjects' breath following absorption through the skin (8).

In other words, the essential oils penetrate into the skin, make it into the bloodstream, diffuse all around the body to various organs including the lungs and are then breathed out. Eventually they are excreted through the kidneys in the urine, exhaled by the lungs, secreted through the skin or passed through in the feces.

Topical application of essential oils can be used for therapeutic purposes, like healing a cut or burn; in skincare to help cell regeneration; in massages for calming or invigorating effects, or help bolster the immune system; or on compresses to help with inflammation.

HOW LONG ARE THE ESSENTIAL OILS ACTIVE AND EFFECTIVE? WHAT IS BIOAVAILABILITY WHEN INHALED AND WHEN APPLIED TOPICALLY?

First, the answer of how long essential oils are active depends on whether they are inhaled or used topically. Dr. Joie Powers discussed averages and general effectiveness in a recent NAHA (National Association of Holistic Aromatherapists) talk (9).

Bioavailability: bioavailability is the proportion of substance introduced into the body able to have an active effect. However, no two people will handle bioavailability of the same substance in exactly the same way. Age, skin condition, diet, blood circulation, general health, body temperature, room temperature and other factors all play into this – as well as the concentration of the essential oil used.

In general, the only 100% bioavailability is when a substance is injected. Essential oils:

+ When inhaled – bioavailability with essential oils can be 70%

+ Compare this to an oral drug like morphine with only 23.9% bioavailability
(any drug swallowed, that goes through the stomach and processed by the liver typically has a lower bioavailability)

+ When topically applied (depending on whether neat or diluted),
bioavailability of essential oils is generally about 7%.

<u>However consider the "peak concession" or "half-life"</u>

(that is, when half of the essential oil has reached its effective peak and will start to wane)

+ When applied topically – peak concession is 360 minutes

+ When inhaled – peak concession is 20 minutes

+ When combined inhale and topical – peak concession is 20 minutes

(inhalation trumps the speed and percentage of bioavailability, but the EO will linger longer due to topical application).

Tisserand & Young note a number of studies that indicate once an essential oil has been absorbed by the skin, the epidermis may act as a reservoir, retaining some of the EO for up to 72 hours but the majority is absorbed in 24 hours. One study noted: tea tree oil was applied to the skin, 2.75% of the dose crossed the epidermis and 0.3% was retained after 24 hours. (10)

Even though bioavailability is low when used topically only, we recommend that most usages should combine inhalation AND topical for a fuller, more effective result. And even though bioavailability is lower when applied topically, if using an essential oil for a therapeutic purpose that would benefit a longer, slower action (healing a burn or cut, antiaging skincare, inflammation, fungal treatment, acne treatment, etc.), it may be a beneficial effect. One would reapply the oil or blend again, and also inhale again in this case.

A WORD ON ORAL DOSING

I don't recommend experimenting with ingestion, as mentioned earlier. Some certified aromatherapists or doctors may recommend oral ingestion under their supervision and this is preferred, typically for a serious disease or infection.

Some in the general public might add a drop of essential oils to their beverage, as a personal choice. But you should realize that stomach acids may break down the components, and certainly the EO will pass to the liver, where a significant portion could be deactivated – or in a few cases, made more toxic.

Know also that there is a risk of agitating stomach lining and mucosa (more sensitive than skin.) Newbies, please don't experiment. Rely on those trained in the pharmacology and science of constituents, and certified in essential oils.

I tend to agree with Dr. Joie Powers who reminds us use of essential oils is called aromatherapy for a reason! Inhaling is the most powerful and beneficial, as demonstrated in this book.

Now back to inhalation and topical uses…

Remember the purpose and use of your essential oils as well: sometimes you are diffusing just to purify the air and | or to create an inviting environment. This application is different than using an essential oil to treat a cut, burn or inflammation, for instance.

Robert Tisserand and Rodney Young PhD write on the subject of essential oil absorption in the body systems well and also chart the information Dr. Powers discussed, so if you are interested in this subject, be sure to pick up the book. "Essential Oil Safety, A Guide for Healthcare Professionals" published by Churchill Livingstone, 2nd edition 2014.

THE IMMUNE SYSTEM AND ESSENTIAL OILS

A number of essential oils have the power to support immune system functions. When you have a strong immune system, you are less likely to get ill or are able to fight illness more effectively and be sick less often.

Because essential oils are able to kill fungus, bacteria, virus and microbes; because they can help boost white blood cells and boost circulation; because they can help with oxygenation and stimulate the immune system; because they can help reduce stress and pain, which is a burden on the immune system; essential oils are our immune system allies.

It's important to understand how your immune system works, and how your overall health can be affected. You are actually born with basic immunity against disease, partly from the healthy bacteria residing in your intestines, on your skin, and in the mucosa (known as the microbiome). These bacteria help protect against invaders, but if they are impaired or fail, other immune cells can take up the fight, and then your lymphatic system and organs step up. Scientists say the immune system develops a kind of memory against the invader once conquered.

However, if your immune system is worn down, overloaded or weakened, it has a harder time fighting off infections and microbes. Factors that hurt the immune system include stress, lack of sleep, poor diet (which may hurt the good bacteria in the gut), no exercise, poor circulation, negative mood, taking in too many toxins, etc.

Keep your immune system strong to stay well. Essential oils can help.

- ✓ Some essential oils help build up white blood cells, like bergamot, eucalyptus, Roman chamomile, lavender, lemon, myrrh, Siberian pine needle, sandalwood, tea tree, thyme and vetiver.

- ✓ Some help boost blood circulation that feeds the body and delivers nutrients, like cinnamon leaf, geranium, peppermint, eucalyptus and ginger.

- ✓ Others increase immune activity (immune stimulants) like clove, cinnamon leaf, eucalyptus globulus, frankincense, turmeric, oregano and sage.

✓ Some bring down stress (including cortisol levels) and help support the immune system, like rose geranium, rosemary, lavender, frankincense, tea tree, clary sage and ylang ylang.

THE IMMUNE SYSTEM IS AFFECTED BY EMOTIONAL MOOD, TOO

Overall wellness, both emotional and physical, affects the immune system. In other words, being stressed, sad or negative can have an impact on the immune system as much as physical stress, poor diet, being worn down or exposed to microbes. A strong immune system is the ideal for vibrant health.

Dr. Mercola writes about different kinds of stress affecting different aspects of the immune system.

Brief stress, such as making a speech or taking a test, tends to suppress cellular immunity (acquired immunity mediated by antigen-specific T-cell lymphosites; involved in resistance to infectious diseases) while preserving humoral immunity (which refers to antibody production and accompanying processes). As a result, you may find yourself more vulnerable to the common cold or flu.

Chronic stress, such as caring every day for a partner or parent with dementia, suppresses both components of the immune system, making you more susceptible not just to infectious diseases, but all disease. (11)

Building a strong immune system or maintaining one (and supporting the lymphatic system) is absolutely key. I am a fan of daily Dry Skin Brushing to support the lymphatic system, and because it invigorates the body and spirit.

I equally support daily Oil Pulling because it help draws out bacteria and microbes from the mouth that the lymphatic system won't have to deal with, and promotes healthy oral health which is linked to overall body wellness and the immune system. (I sometimes put a drop of an essential oil in the organic oil before Oil Pulling)

Of course, exercise, a balanced diet, lots of fresh water and other healthy habits also contribute to a good immune system.

Essential oils have their role to play in this. A number of essential oils have been shown to support and boost the immune system. We have just name a number of them and if we were to name the most effective overall, they would be: Cinnamon, Clove, Sage, Thyme, Lemon, Oregano, Rosemary and Frankincense.

PSYCHONEUROIMMUNOLOGY

The immune system is actually quite complex, working with the lymphatic system to "cleanse and draw out" toxins in the system and help strengthen the body. There is also impact on the brain, found in the new science of Psychoneuroimmunology.

Medical News Today reports that the intriguing links between neuroscience and the immune system are slowly being uncovered and studied in this new interdisciplinary area of study called Psychoneuroimmunology. (12)

The brain exerts its power on the immune system through chemical messengers in reaction to something the brain perceives. For instance, when stressed or frightened, the brain (limbic system) sends cortisol into the system. The brain (hypothalamus) regulates temperate, blood sugar levels and hormones which affect the immune system.

As explained by Dr. Joie Power, PhD (13), the connections between the hypothalamus and the immune system are bi-directional: the brain not only transmits information to the immune system but receives information from it! It is the way in which states of mind influence the body and the body influences the mind.

We will explore more of this particular subject in Chapter 6 Mind-Body-Spirit. But before we go any further into the subject of what essential oils do, let's examine their history – as it will put a perspective on everything!

Chapter 2

FASCINATING HISTORY: AROMATIC PLANTS TO ESSENTIAL OILS

There is no substitute for cultivating an understanding of the natural way our soul and body works and how that precious natural balance can be maintained.
~ Kurt Schnaubelt, Ph.D.

If you enjoy short podcasts about history & essential oils, you'll love this episode of Essential Oil Zen entitled Kings and Queens and Lavender!

Let's set the stage for the rest of the book, giving you context on the long history of aromatic plants and essential oils.

Aromatic plants and essential oils have been used for thousands and thousands of years. People have long valued fragrances for their spiritual and physical cleansing, and pleasurable effects plus health applications.

I love history and understanding how things came to be or were developed over time. (My Bachelor's degree was in art history in Paris, which pulled together art, politics, religion, science, economics and lifestyle of each era.) When I started studying the history of essential oils, I typically found a paragraph to a page stating that essential oils were first used in Ancient Egypt; mention of Ancient Greece and Rome; and then zoom forward to the early 1900's and René-Maurice Gattefossé, considered the father of "modern" aromatherapy – he coined the term and devoted his life to its study in the south of France.

I wanted to go deeper into the history of essential oils, and indeed found really interesting facts to share with you!

The first thing to state: essential oils as we use them today were not as such until steam distillation was "invented". Susruta, an Ayurvedic master in the 2nd century, described in the Book of Ayurveda how to obtain rose oil, citronella oil and calamus by distillation.(1) Ancient Egyptians were familiar with fire and the distillation process, producing turpentine, for instance.

There is evidence of crude distillation apparati at several archaeological sites and in a few museums (Cyprus, Iraq, what is now Syria and elsewhere) dating prior to ancient Egypt. Aromatic plants and infused waters or the aromatic essences in fat-soluble solutions were certainly used with beneficial results.

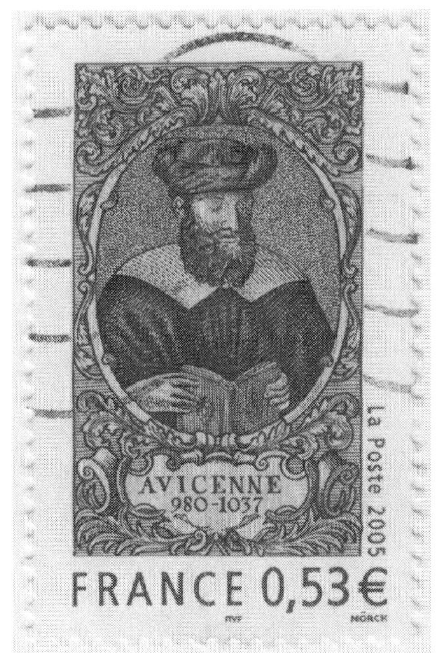

However, the first more modern documented proof of steam distillation machinery came with the brilliant Avicenna (10th century) – you'll read more about him in this chapter. So, while frankincense, peppermint and myrrh are valued just as much today as they were centuries ago when mentioned in various texts, they were just in a slightly different "format" than in our more modern era.

The roots and history of aromatherapy is believed to have begun with the burning of fragrant woods, leaves, needles, and tree gums. The first evidence of early humans using fire dates back to more than a million years, but the practice did not become routine until about 650,000 years later.

This practice of burning fragrant plants probably arose once it was discovered that when burning certain plants, such as cypress and cedar, scents filled the air and perhaps some change of mood or even wellness effects were felt or discovered. (Of course, this is speculation on my part but it seems logical.)

We do know that plants were viewed as powerful, considered to have magical attributes and were employed in various ceremonies, applications and healing rituals to appease the spirits and combat curses (2)

The earliest evidence of human knowledge of the

healing properties of plants was found in Lascaux, located in the Dordogne region in France (France again!). There, cave paintings suggest the use of medicinal plants in everyday life that have been carbon dated as far back as 18,000 B.C.

The archeological evidence for medicinal use of plants (including oils) by humans in the areas that are now Texas and northeastern Mexico extends back 10,500 years ago. Psychoactive plants have a long history of use in the form of smoke for ritual and medicinal purposes - the early precursors of aromatherapy. In many cultures, plant smoke is still widely used in cleansing rituals and is believed to carry messages to the spirit world. That very same belief is behind the burning of frankincense in Catholic churches.

Ancient written records (clay tablets) documenting the medicinal use of plants come to us from the ancient Sumerians, who lived in Mesopotamia from about 5,500 B.C. Sumeria is often referred to as the cradle of civilization (along with Akkad and Babylon). Aromatic essences were quite highly prized with the

Sumerians. The written records actually detail what they used, how they prepared the plants or oils and dosages.

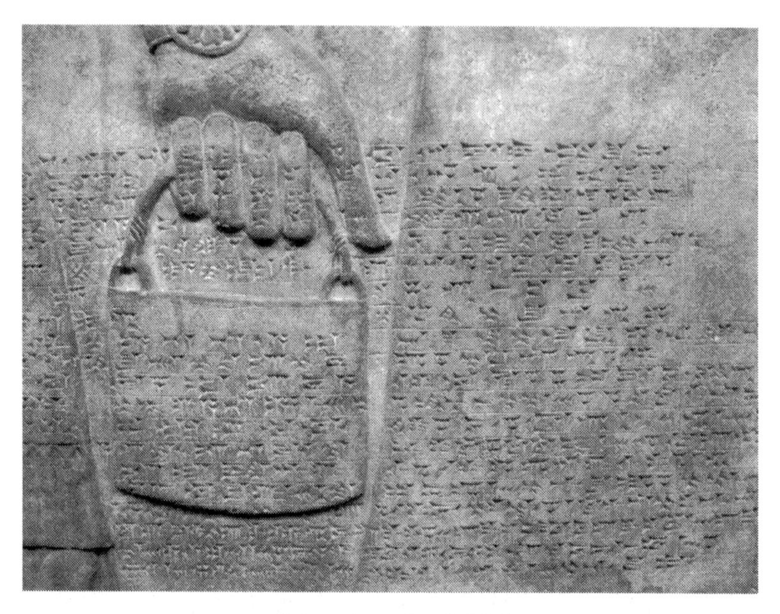

Sumerian clay tablet

In Sumeria, clay pots were filled with plant material which was then covered in water; an absorbent cloth of some kind was stuffed into the opening and the pot heated. As the water turned to steam and rose towards the opening of the jar, the essential oils were trapped in the material, which could then be wrung out to produce a mixture of water and essential oils that would have been similar to today's hydrosols.

Myrrh is mentioned in one of the oldest epics, the Gilgamesh from Mesopotamia, in which Ut-napitschti, the urfather thanks God for his salvation from the Deluge by burning cedarwood and myrrh.

The Babylonians, who lived in the same general area from about 3000 B.C. to 600 B.C. also left records detailing the use of medicinal herbs and plants. The Assyrians followed the Babylonians in about 628 B.C. They not only preserved the clay tablets of the earlier civilizations, but left their own. They believed that disease was largely considered to be the work of evil spirits or demons (a belief that passed through many eras). The most common way of ridding themselves of these demons was smoking them out with fragrant plants. Mentioned in the various texts were chamomile, myrrh, turmeric and calendula.

I found it exciting that there was an enormous trade in aromatic plants in the ancient world. The Babylonians imported frankincense from Africa and burned about 57,000 pounds of it a year. The Assyrians burned about 120,000 pounds of it a year in their annual feast of Baal. In fact, Babylon became the center of the aromatics trade in the late 5th century B.C. and among the most common plants they used were cypress, pine, fir, myrtle, frankincense, calamus and juniper.

ANCIENT EGYPTIANS

The Egyptians are probably most famous for their use of aromatic plants and oils. They made extensive use of resins, dried plants, infused oils and pomades. Fragrant plants were used for embalming, for religious rituals, for diffusing in living spaces and for healing; it is known they commonly used cedar, myrrh, and frankincense among others.

The earliest historical accounts of the Egyptian use of aromatics date to about 4,500 B.C. - about 1000 years after the Sumerians. However, the most famous historical document describing the use of aromatic medicine by the Egyptians is the Ebers Papyrus, (found near Thebes in 1872.) The Ebers Papyrus was written during the reign of Khufu, around 2800 B.C., and describes the use of over 850 botanical remedies

including myrrh, frankincense, myrtle, galbanum and many other aromatic herbs. The use of myrrh as a wound salve is mentioned specifically.
Gattefossé wrote in his book that embalming dates back beyond ancient Egypt (they just perfected it) to the Copper Age or beginning of the Bronze Age. (3). He further wrote that many ancient rites used essential oils or spices, burned in their natural state (like juniper, rosemary). The aromatics created an emotional atmosphere but the holy sites like temples were seen as very healthy and pure, too. The essential oils or aromatic plants were of course overcoming microbes and bacteria.

Ancient Egyptians used incense, essential oils, infused waters, ointments and resins for various religious ceremonies. They used frankincense on a large scale, burning it for purification in sacred spaces and for use in the pharaoh's living spaces. It is said that terra cotta urns filled with aromatic essential oils accompanied the pharaohs to the afterlife. Oils of cedarwood, clove, cinnamon, nutmeg and myrrh were used to embalm the dead (discovered in some tombs that were opened in this century. It was reported that some light scents of various oils remained at discovery!)

King Tutankhamun was entombed with roughly 350 liters of aromatic oil including cedarwood, frankincense, and myrrh.

In 1370 BC, Pharoah Amenophis IV, husband of Nefertiti, received a request from Milkili, one of his military lieutenants serving in Palestine saying, "And let the King, my Lord, send troops to his servants, and let the King, my Lord, send myrrh for medicine." It was said that he refused to fight until the physicians with his troops had a good supply of myrrh . (4)

In art history classes, I learned that Egyptian men of the time used fragrance as much as the women. An interesting method used (seen in tomb art) was to place a solid waxy cone of perfume on their heads (as seen here). It would gradually melt and cover them in fragrance.

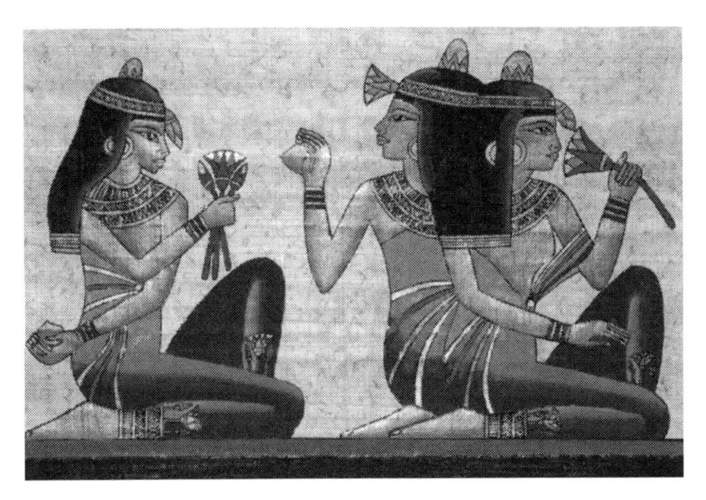

It is reported that Queen Hatshepsut's expedition to the legendary land of Punt (about 1470 B.C.) was a truly great adventure of antiquity. Her army brought back wondrous riches - the greatest of all the treasures was a grove of myrrh trees.

By 500 B.C. the Nile Valley was considered the 'Cradle of Medicine' because of its expert use of oils and herbs for healing.

Queen Cleopatra kept massive gardens of hundreds of flowers and used their essences to perfume her body and surroundings. Both the Queen of Sheba and Cleopatra loved lavender for various purposes (including seducing lovers, it is said!)

AYURVEDIC INDIA

During the time when Egyptians were using plants and oils for perfumes, incense, and embalming, early healers in India developed the Ayurvedic system of medicine - the oldest form of medicine. Ayurveda is from ayur "life" + veda "knowledge" and is based on the idea of balance in bodily systems and uses diet, herbal treatment, and yogic breathing.

"Ayurvedic practices include the use of herbal medicines, mineral or metal supplementation (rasa shastra), surgical techniques, opium, and application of oil by massages." (5)

A portion of the Rig Veda written around 4,500 BC records the use of aromatic herbs. As mentioned at the beginning of the Chapter, the Book of Ayurveda and Susruta included information about essential oil use and its application in the 2nd century.

CHINA

Legendary Chinese ruler Shen Nung is credited with discovering the medicinal properties of plants and writing the first herbal text, 'Pen Tsao' (c. 2700-3000

B.C.), which is a catalog of more than 200 botanicals. The first herbal of Chinese medicine, written in the second century, also known as Shen Nung Ben Cao, classifies plants in the categories of prevention, restorative and treatment. It addresses the jing (essence) of plants, corresponding to our understanding of essential oils. The Chinese 'Yellow Emperor's Classic of Internal Medicine', was written in 2697 B.C. and is the oldest surviving medical book in China.

ANCIENT GREECE AND ROME

The ancient Greeks used an array of essential oils. We know they used lavender to fight insomnia, insanity and some pains like back aches. Greek soldiers carried myrrh into battle with them to use for skin infections, cuts and gangrene.

After Alexander's invasion of Egypt in the 3rd century B.C., the use of aromatics, herbs and perfumes became much more popular in Greece prompting great interest in all things aromatic!

The wonderful Greek physician Hippocrates (460 to 375 B.C.) is considered the father of modern medicine. It is said that he used essential oils for baths and purification for medicinal purposes. Historical records showed he fumigated Athens with plant aromatics saving many from a plague.

Theophrastus of Athens, who was a philosopher and student of Aristotle, investigated everything about plants and even how scents affected the emotions. He wrote several volumes on botany including 'The History of Plants', which became a top botanical science reference for centuries to come. He is generally referred to today as the "Founder of Botany".

Between 300 B.C. and 100 B.C. Persian traders brought myrrh and frankincense from Yemen to the Mediterranean, especially Greece and Rome, and soon demand grew for roses, saffron, spikenard, ginger and many other aromatics. The first century AD was a time of great progress for aromatherapy. About 2,800 tons of Frankincense was imported to Rome per year during this era, and Pliny's book, "Natural

History", includes 32 flower remedies. (6)

A Greek perfumer by the name of Megallus created a perfume called "megaleion" which became quite popular and well-used. Megaleion included myrrh in a fatty-oil base and served several purposes: (a) as a perfume, (b) as an anti-inflammatory remedy for the skin and (c) as a product to heal wounds. It included myrrh and cinnamon.

Pliny the Elder (23-79 A.D.) described a widely used essential oil blend called kyphi. It included cypress, juniper, frankincense, myrrh, calamus and other aromatics mixed with honey. Kyphi was used for medical purposes and in worship. Dioscordes wrote that kyphi brought relaxation, promoted sleep and calm. The Roman historian and botanist Pliny the Elder also recommended frankincense as an antidote to hemlock poisoning, and wrote in the first century A.D. that this amazing resin had made the southern Arabians the richest people on earth.

Pedanius Dioscordes (30-90 A.D.) had a passion for plants, and catalogued all the known herbs and their uses in his enormous work, “De Materia Medica” (five volumes) in 70 A.D. Dioscordes was born in Turkey and became a traveling physician, even traveling with Nero’s army. Most of his works were written in Greek, and they became known by many, and then translated into many languages. To make a comparison as far as the depth of what Dioscordes did: everything Hippocrates wrote on medicinal plants totals about 130 articles. Dioscordes listed over 4,740 different uses in his book, and lists more than 360 varieties of medicinal actions.

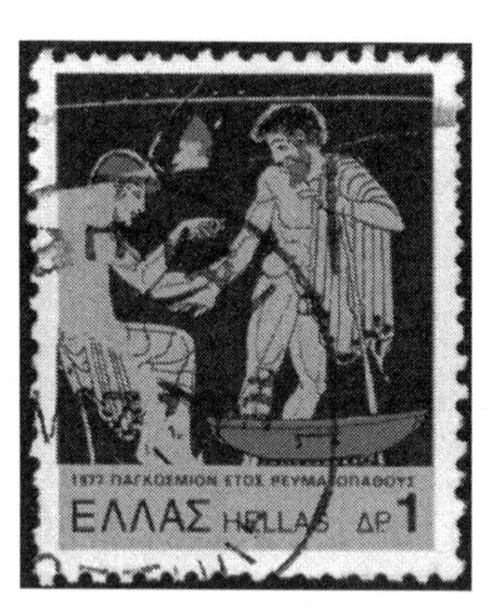

He took a very scientific approach: Dioscorides didn't accept anything on faith or “hear-say”, or on the reputation of established authorities; he checked everything out himself that he included in his books, and tested every drug clinically. He personally traveled and researched the local folk medicine uses of every herb he wrote about.

Another brilliant Greek physician was Claudius Galen, who lived from 129-199 A.D. and studied medicine from the age of seventeen. He began his medical career at age 28 under the Romans, treating wounds of gladiators with medicinal herbs - and it is said that not a single gladiator died of battle wounds while under his care.

Roman soldiers treated wounds with honey and myrrh, while emperors and scholars relaxed in legendary perfumed baths. Romans loved using lavender in the public baths. In both Greece and Rome, Myrrh was used as a remedy for skin sores, for treating mouth and eye infections, as a cough remedy, against worm infestation and even for cattle abdominal pains.

Due to his phenomenal success, Galen quickly rose to become the personal physician to the Roman Emperor, Marcus Aurelius, and since Rome was a thriving academic center during his lifetime, it was the ideal place to conduct further research. Galen was the last of the great Greco-Roman physicians, and within 100 years of his death the Roman Empire would begin to decline, plunging Europe into the dark ages.

Suzanne Bovenizer CMT, CST, writes about the Romans (7):

> *The Romans took the use of essential oils to new extremes. In self-indulgent Rome, lavish baths were created as focal points for Roman life. Men would gather in the mid afternoon at these communal bathing facilities and not only soak in water, but compete in sports like wrestling, have business meetings, wander through gardens and enjoy entertainment. Before the sports, men would be oiled up usually with olive oil, then have their bodies scraped with a curved metal wire to take off excess dirt and sweat. Plunges into a variety of bathes from cool to hot were followed with massages rich in fragrant unguents.*
>
> *There were 3 main types of perfumes used at this time: "Ladysmata" were solid unguents, "Stymmata" were scented oils, and "Diapasmata" were powdered perfumes. Recipes for favorite aromatics used during this*

period were archived. One was called "Susinum" which was a combination of honey, calamus, cinnamon, myrrh, and saffron. "Nardinum" brought together calamus, costus, cardamom, melissa, spikenard and myrrh. These would be used in cosmetics, or in massage, rubbed on hair, or even scented bed clothes. One interesting note was that the scent of orange was reserved only for courtesans and ladies of a similar trade, which if you think of the aphrodisiac qualities of neroli, you can imagine why... As stated earlier, men enjoyed smelling as sweetly as women. Although women were allowed to use the bathes, they had to pay more and usually met only in the mornings, staying segregated from the men.By 3 AD, Rome was the bathing capital of Europe, with 1,000 fragrant spas in the city alone. Nero, the then debauched, self-serving emperor, lavished himself in scented bliss, particularly taking pleasure in the scent of roses, believing that the oil not only uplifted spirits, but also helped with headaches and indigestion. One would drink out of perfumed cups and walk through spice-

scented rooms when visiting Nero's palace. Unguents were being so widely used by that point in history, that in 30 AD supplies of exotic plants and herbs were becoming scarce. An edict was drafted encouraging less personal use of aromatics so that the supplies could be used more for medicinal, religious and ritual purposes.(7)

BIBLICAL TIMES

Around 1200 B.C., the Book of Exodus records how the Jews took too much knowledge of herbs and spices with them as they fled from Egypt. A recipe for an anointing oil was given to Moses (blending myrrh, cinnamon, calamus and olive oils 500-400 B.C.)

The Old and New Testaments of the Bible contain recipes using aromatic compounds – there are more than 500 references to Essential Oils (especially frankincense and myrrh and spikenard, part of the valerian family.) The wise men, as we know, brought the valuable gift of frankincense and myrrh to the birth of Jesus – they were considered as valuable as gold.

Mary used lavender to anoint Jesus' feet.

THRIVING EARLY PERSIA

Al-Razi (865-925) is considered one of Persia's finest physicians. Like many intellectuals in his day, he lived at various small courts under the patronage of minor rulers. During his lifetime he wrote more than 237 books and articles covering several fields of science, half of which concerned medicine. Quite a few were translated into Latin. Born in the town of Rayy near Tehran, Al-Razi was known in the West as Rhazes where he had great influence on European science and medicine.

His most influential work was a medical encyclopedia covering 25 books called "Al Kitab al Hawi", which was later translated into Latin and other European languages, and known in English as "The Comprehensive Work".

His medical accomplishments were legendary. This man was quite amazing - he developed such things as spatulas, mortars, and flasks used in pharmacies for centuries (until the 1900s).

In the 10th century, the well-known Persian philosopher, child genius, physician and scientist Avicenna (980 to 1037) “invented” and used the first steam distillation for essential oils, later refined during the Renaissance in western Europe. Avicenna invented a coiled pipe which allowed the plant vapor and steam to cool down more effectively than previous distillers that used a straight cooling pipe. Avicenna's contribution led to more focus on essential oils and their benefits in the years that followed.

At the age of 16 Avicenna began studying medicine and by 20 he had been appointed a court physician, earning the title 'Prince of Physicians'. He wrote books covering theology, metaphysics, astronomy, philology, philosophy and poetry, and most influentially, 20 books and 100 treatises on medicine.
His 14 volume epic “Al-Qanun fi al-Tibb”, which means “The Canon of Medicine” was over one million words long. It included the total of what was known to that day of existing medical knowledge, including Galen and Hippocrates and other eminent figures who preceded him.

Anecdote: when the sultan of Bukhara became ill and the court physicians couldn't figure it out or help him, Avicenna was called to his bedside - and cured him. This earned him the gratitude of the sultan, who opened the royal Sāmānid library to him. This was an amazing gift, giving him access to much knowledge and written works on medicine and science.

Another anecdote: Avicenna excelled at the preparation of rose water (a favored plant of Persians) and other infused oil waters by blowing live steam into the distillation vessel filled with plants. Thus, it seems relatively certain that Avicenna invented a more modern process of steam distillation.

MEDIEVAL TIMES TO THE RENAISSANCE IN WESTERN EUROPE

As the Romans began pulling out of Britain and Europe, much of their vast medical knowledge that had been collected and passed from Greece, ancient Egypt, Persia and other enlightened places was all but discarded. All progress in the Western tradition of medicine came to a halt for hundreds of years, in a time appropriately nicknamed "The Dark Ages."

The oldest surviving English manuscript of botanical medicine is the Saxon "Leech Book of Bald", which was written between 900 and 950 by a scribe named Cild under the direction of Bald, who was a friend of King Alfred the Great. ("Leech" is an old English word meaning healer). This book includes descriptions of 500 plants and how they could be used internally or externally. In addition to herbalism, it includes magic, shamanism and ceremonial rites.

Interestingly, as recently reported by the BBC (March 2015) on antibiotic resistant bacteria, the "Leech Book of Bald" and a specific recipe were cited:

"Scientists recreated a 9th Century Anglo-Saxon remedy using onion, garlic and part of a cow's stomach. They were "astonished" to find it almost completely wiped out methicillin-resistant staphylococcus aureus, otherwise known as MRSA. Their findings will be presented at a national microbiology conference ...Anglo-Saxon expert Dr. Christina Lee, from the University of Nottingham, translated the recipe...Experts from the university's microbiology team recreated the remedy and then tested it on large cultures of MRSA ... In each case, they tested the individual ingredients against the bacteria, as well as the remedy and a control solution.

They found the remedy killed up to 90% of MRSA bacteria and believe it is the effect of the recipe rather than one single ingredient." (8)

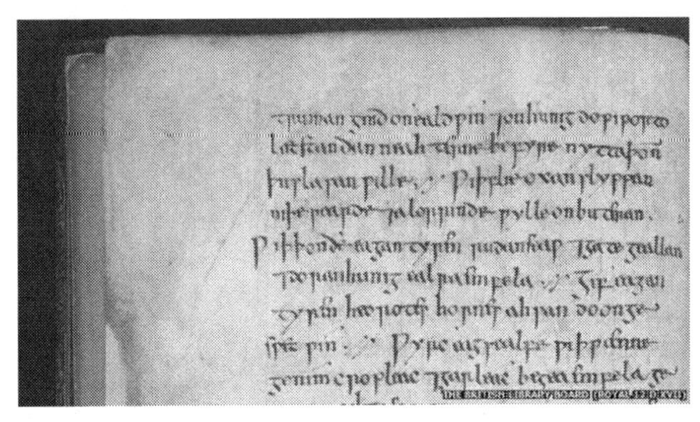

courtesy British Library: Leech Book of Bald

When the Crusaders returned from the Holy Wars (1095-1291), they brought with them aromatic plants, perfumes and healing remedies that were previously unknown or had been discarded centuries prior. Fragrant plants became popular, with aromatic herb garlands decorating homes and rose water being used to wash the hands of those who could afford it.

The availability and range of aromatic medicines continued to increase over the next few hundred years.

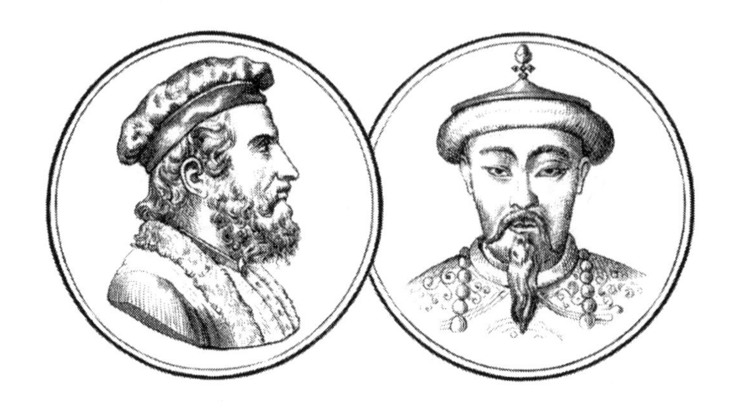

Marco Polo and Kubla Khan

With Marco Polo (1254-1324), the much-prized spices and aromatics of India, China, and beyond sparked European trade and renewed interest. Spices and oils such as cardamom, sage, cinnamon, and nutmeg were reintroduced, and pharmacists (such as they were in the era) began to work with the imports more.

In the 12th century, Hildegard, an Abbess of Germany, is said to have grown and distilled lavender for its medicinal properties. The iconic Cathedral in Santiago de Compostelo (Spain), where pilgrimages were led year after year since Medieval times (think "Canterbury Tales"), has the largest Frankincense burner in the world.

The "Red Book of Hergest" is a large vellum manuscript written shortly after 1382 in Wales. It ranks as one of the most important medieval manuscripts written in the Welsh language. Not only is there poetry and historical stories, but it also includes herbal remedies. These were associated with Rhiwallon Feddyg, founder of a medical dynasty in Wales that lasted over 500 years. 'The Physicians of Myddfai were from the village of Myddfai - this text is being reexamined again today for secrets and research into essential oils.

The horrid Black Death appeared in the 14th century (around 1347), killing millions of people across Europe. It was devastating. Almost 50% of London's inhabitants succumbed within the first year, and up to 40% of the entire population of Europe would die within 3 years.

In Europe at that time, medicine was almost entirely

governed by the Catholic Church. The church considered illness and disease to be a punishment from God or even demons incarnate, and the standard form of treatment administered by the priests was prayer, and perhaps a session of blood-letting. The Church rejected "pagan fragrances" because they stimulated forbidden instincts or heightened pleasure. The church saw physicians and their plants and oils as competition for curing mind and soul as well as unreligious. Sigh.

Historical anecdote: During the plague in France (around 1400 A.D.), four thieves in Marseilles were robbing the unfortunate dead – without becoming sick. When they were eventually caught, their secret was revealed: they used a blend of essential oils and aromatics to protect themselves from getting sick. The blend included cinnamon, rosemary, clove, eucalyptus and lemon. Today, there are essential oil blends called Thieves or Four Thieves, in memory of the event.

In fact, during this period perfumers and tanners in England and France escaped the Plague, too, due to the overwhelming amounts of aromatic plans and essential oils they used which passed on the antibacterial qualities.

Moufitte, a writer during the period, noted in his book "Treatise on Food" that an entire town in England called Bucklersbury was "replete" with spices and oils. Being so perfumed in the time of the plague, it escaped as multitudes died in the next towns away. In Shakespeare's "The Merry Wives of Windsor", Falstaff makes a reference to the aromatic Bucklersbury: "Come, I cannot cog, and say thou art this and that like many of these lisping hawthorn buds, that come like women in men's apparel, and smell like Bucklersbury in simple time." Bucklersbury was the center of the European Lavender trade.

Despite the Church forbidding aromatic oils, herbal preparations were used to help fight this terrible killer. It is believed that some perfumers and herbalists may have avoided the plague due to their continual contact with essential oils and plants (with anti-bacterial and cleansing power.)

Certainly, when the Black Death made its second

appearance in 1603, virtually every available aromatic was burned in houses and on the streets to help keep the plaque at bay. Benzoin, frankincense and various spice oils were all used to prevent the spread of this deadly disease. The only people not to succumb in large numbers to the plague (both times) were the workers involved in aromatics and perfumery, and this is undoubtedly due to the highly antiseptic properties of the essential oils.

RENAISSANCE

The Renaissance revitalized everything in European society, including aromatherapy with imports from the East; explorer merchants brought back exotic herbs and oils. With the Renaissance and certainly by the 15th century, things were evolving more quickly. More plants were distilled to create essential oils including frankincense, juniper, rose, sage and rosemary. A growth in the amount of books on herbs and their properties also begins later in the century.

Herbal medicine was used by all, from peasants to kings. King Henry VIII (born 1491) was a huge advocate of herbal medicine and as well as treatment from his own apothecaries, even enjoyed making his own remedies. His charter of 1543 gave herbalists the right to practice (although it was taken away later). Records show that Tudors in Henry VIII's time treated headaches by drinking a mixture of lavender, sage, marjoram, rose and rue, as just one example.

Paracelsus (1493-1541) was an alchemist, author, teacher, medical doctor and philosopher born near Zurich. He is credited with coining the term "Essence" for essential oils, and his studies radically challenged the nature of alchemy as he focused upon using plants as medicines. He moved away from the medical applications of his day which included bleeding and purging; he travelled widely and gathered information. However, he incurred the wrath of many with his eccentric character, and by rejecting Galen and Avicenna. (9)

In 1564, the authors Charles Estienne and Jean Liebaul wrote in L'Agriculture et Maison Rustique: "Distilled oils are found by experience to be more valid, more efficacious, more pleasant, and of more rapid effect than any other, to cure all kinds of difficult diseases, especially wounds, ulcers…" (10)

Of note, around this time (about 1500 A.D.), Spanish Conquistadors invaded the Aztecs, and were amazed to find an abundance of aromatic, medicinal herbs in Montezuma's garden and knowledge of its use.

Queen Elizabeth I (1533-1603), the daughter of Henri VIII, used an abundant supply of English lavender oil throughout her life, a practice continued by Queen Victoria during her entire 64-year reign. (The tradition was upheld in the 20th century by Diana, Princess of Wales, who regularly visited her aromatherapist. It is known that her living quarters were usually fragrant with various essential oils.)

A German physician, Hieronymus Braunschweig, wrote several books on essential oil distillation which went through hundreds of editions in every European language at the time. In 1597 he referenced 25 essential oils included rosemary, lavender, clove, cinnamon, myrrh, and nutmeg.

Many books about distillation of essential oils were written in the 16th century, especially in Germany, which seemed to be one of the centers of an aromatherapy renaissance.

Several English sources from the 1500s and 1600s give detailed recipes for sweet waters and for distilling essential oils, such as Gervase Markham's 1615 “English Housewife”, John French's 1653 “Art of Distillation”, and Hugh Plat's 1594 “Delightes for Ladies”. Many (modern or contemporary) sources claim that the oldest alcohol based perfumes were Queen of Hungary Water (a rosemary-based water) and Carmelite water (or King Charles' water), whose ingredients vary-- both allegedly “invented” in the late 1300s and originally used as medicinal doses and rubs.

During the 16th century, one could buy oils at an "apothecary," and many more essential oils were introduced, thanks to growing trade and interested populace. This widespread use of essential oils throughout Europe coincided with the invention of glass distillation methods in the 16th century, the discovery of new trade routes east and the invention of the microscope, which facilitated the study of bio-active compounds. And in fact, in the 16th century, there were comprehensive plant catalogs available. Anyone who could read had access to recipes for oils, perfumed waters and other methods of treating plants for wellness. Advancements in distillation techniques were made in Germany during the 16th century.

Shakespeare wrote in Hamlet (said by Orphelia): "There's rosemary that's for remembrance", acknowledging the power of that essential oil or herb on memory and focus, proven out through researchers today.

Nicholas Culpepper (1616-1654) was one of the most influential herbalists of his time. In his most famous work, "The English Physician" (1652), Culpeper's descriptions of herbs, oils and their uses were intermixed with astrology. It should be noted that in the 17th century, Nicholas Culpeper wrote passionate works against doctors who were using and prescribing poisonous substances such as mercury on patients. (11)

The first and earliest industrial essential oil manufacturers appear in Europe from 1768, according to "Handbook of Essential Oils: Science, Technology, and Applications" edited by K. Husnu Can Baser and Gerhard Buchbauer. These early manufacturers include:

Antoine Chiris (1768) in Grasse, France; Cavallier Freres (1784) in Grasse, France; Dodge & Alcott (1798) in New York (*listed as importers*); Roure Bertrand Fils et Justin Dupont (1820) in Grasse, France; Schimmel & Co (1829) in Leipzig, Germany; M. Mero-Boyveau (1832) in Grasse, France; Standford, Allen & Sons (1833) London; Robertet et Cie (1850) in Grasse, France; and W.J. Bush (1851) London.

Grasse in the south of France has always been an area of aromatic plants, lavender, perfumeries and such. For the New York importers, I tried to track down more information on Dodge & Alcott and didn't get far. They seemed to favor importing perfumes.

19TH CENTURY FORWARD

American companies began manufacturing products with essential oils, like soaps and perfumes. Most of this industry was located in New York, with its access to imported spices, aromatics and French fragrances. As far as essential oils, it seemed the emphasis was more on household products and synthetic products rather than a large-scale population recognizing them for healing, as in Europe and the East.

There were holistic, homeopath and naturopath movements during this time, of course, with some quite devoted to the new natural movements - and other “traditionalists” who were quite hostile to the movement.

Back in Europe, with the rise of chemistry in the late 19th century, the demystification developed and more availability essential oils developed thanks to the distillation process.

In 1867 a curious thing happened in the world of essential oils. (12) The official concept of "perfume for cosmetics" appeared at the Paris International

Exhibition - "Exposition Universelle". For the first time perfumes, scented gloves, and soaps where clearly displayed separately from medicinal plant essences. The exposition began on April 1, 1867 and closed on October 31, 1867 with over 9,000,000 visitors! This seems to be the beginning of the division of scent for health vs scent just for the sake of scent without regards to health.

RENE-MAURICE GATTEFOSSE

Modern aromatherapy is memorialized and "born" with French chemist Rene-Maurice Gattefossé, who worked for a prominent perfumer in the south of France (Grasse). One day there was a horrible accident in the lab and he set his arm on fire. Contrary to what is found on many websites, Robert Tisserand confirms he DID NOT thrust his arm into the nearest vat of lavender oil willy-nilly. The translation of Gattefossé's own words by Tisserand:

> *"The external application of small quantities of essences rapidly stops the spread of gangrenous sores. In my*

personal experience, after a laboratory explosion covered me with burning substances which I extinguished by rolling on a grassy lawn, both my hands were covered with a rapidly developing gas gangrene. Just one rinse with lavender essence stopped "the gasification of the tissue". This treatment was followed by profuse sweating, and healing began the next day (July 1910)." (13)

His application of lavender oil was clearly an intentional act, not accidental. However, because the results were very impressive, this is a very impactful moment for him and for the history of essential oils and aromatherapy. This was a serious burn and his life had been threatened (gas gangrene was potentially life-threatening.) In addition, previous chemical burns he had received had caused severe pain, redness, blisters and scarring. This bad burn healed with minimal pain and no scarring. And so this incident and discovery of the healing power of lavender began his interest, and then his commitment and lifelong work, with essential oils – to our benefit today!

As was mentioned previously, Gattefossé coined the word "aromatherapie" to describe the healing experience and work with essential oils. He spent the rest of his life researching health benefits of essential oils and collaborating with other doctors and scientists. In 1937, he published his findings and book "Aromatherapie" ("Aromatherapy"). It was translated into English in 1993 by Robert Tisserand and the 2nd edition is still in print, 70 years after it was written (I love my copy and refer to it even today). He is credited with the modern therapeutic approach to holistic healing and balance with essential oils.

French physician Jean Valnet took up and continued the work of Gattefossé during World War II, using chamomile, clove, lemon and thyme essential oils to successfully treat wounded soldiers with gangrene, greatly reducing the need for amputation. After graduating as a surgeon at the end of the war, Valnet continued to use essential oils to treat illnesses, and he was the first ever documented doctor to use them to treat psychiatric conditions. Dr. Valnet recognized the powerful anti-bacterial qualities of essential oils after numerous tests and experiments, and concluded, "Clearly, the administering of essential oils should be common practice in sick rooms, operating rooms and clinics." (14)

During World War II, all Australian soldiers were issued tea tree oil in their first aid kits. The troops used it as an insect repellent and for its fungal-fighting properties.

Historical anecdote, stepping back a decade: With the advent of World War I, the demand for medicine was huge, due to the enormous number of casualties, and herbs were widely used. The garden designer, Gertrude Jekyll set aside a large plot of land just for the growing of Marigolds (Calendula), which was shipped to France to treat burns victims.

Then, during WWII, the British government appealed to the public to help grow herbs for the war effort. In 1940, Whitechapel hospital alerted Kew Gardens that essential supplies of medicines were virtually depleted. Very quickly the Vegetable Drugs

Committee was formed, made up of members of the Ministry of Agriculture and Fisheries, Kew, Pharmaceutical Society and herb growers. Lists of essential plants were drawn up and volunteers helped collect them (including school children and Scouts.) The plants were sold to botanical drug companies to make conventional medicines!

France and active French scientists who were working with essential oils had an influence on the U.K. in this regard.

Valnet's inspired book, 'Aromathérapie - Traitment des Maladies par les Essence de Plantes' (Aromatherapy – Treatment of Illnesses with Essential Oils) was released in 1964. It popularized aromatherapy for medical and psychiatric use throughout France in the 1960s The book was translated into English in 1980, published under the new title of 'The Practice of Aromatherapy', which put aromatherapy squarely on the English map.

Marguerite Maury (1895-1968) was an Austrian-born biochemist who became interested in essential oils, after reading a book written in 1838 by Dr. Chabenes called, "Les Grandes Possibilités par les Matières Odoriferantes". (Dr. Chabenes would become the teacher of Gattefossé.) She published her book in 1962 about the benefits of essential oils, "Le Capital Jeunesse" in France, but sadly did not initially receive the acclaim that it deserved. However, when it was released in Britain in 1964 under the title of "The Secret of Life and Youth", it finally gained recognition.

After her death, the work of Maury continued through her protege, Danièle Ryman, who today is now herself considered an authority on aromatherapy.

The first modern English language book, "The Art of Aromatherapy" by British citizen Robert Tisserand (1977), introduced the benefits of aromatherapy coupled with massage and advanced the practice in the United Kingdom and the United States. Tisserand is a giant in the field of aromatherapy today.

The work of Valnet and Gattefossé stimulated and influenced him. His book became the inspiration and reference for virtually every future author on the subject for almost two decades.

Dr. Paul Belaiche published a three-volume work on the clinical uses of aromatherapy for infectious and degenerative diseases in 1978.

Henri Viaud is also important to mention here in the modern history of aromatherapy. He is a master distiller and led the charge for pure non-unadulterated essential oils that are authentic. Some producers at this time would adulterate oils, but he was firm (and had the voice) that for therapeutic, medicinal value, essential oils must be genuine and pure as distilled.

I will also mention Dr. Kurt Schnaubelt here. He earned his Ph.D in Germany (Technical University of Munich), and has become a leader of aromatherapy in the United States since 1983. He is author of many books on the subject and scientific director of the Pacific Institute of Aromatherapy. He is quoted in this book several times, including on the next pages!

After WWII: Pharma Plus Chemicals

After World War II a huge increase was seen in the production of petrochemicals and synthetics. Production of these chemicals has increased greatly over the years. In 1940 petrochemicals and synthetics were produced at the rate of one billion pounds per year; compare that to 1980 over 400 billion pounds per year were produced (Steinman & Epstein, 1995). Since 1965 more than four million distinct chemical compounds have been reported in scientific literature and of these seventy thousand are used in commercial production. (15)

With the onset of this chemical production “boom”, an increase in health problems has been observed such as asthma and allergies. Other conditions have been noted as well such as headaches, insomnia, reproductive issues and mild depression. This increase of symptoms has been linked to synthetic chemicals and petrochemicals in our environment.

Synthetic offshoots from plants or essential oils? Here are just 2 examples of many: we've cured cold symptoms for generations with Vicks Vaporub, whose main ingredients are synthetic forms of mint (menthol), laurel tree (camphor), and eucalyptus (eucalyptol), in addition to cedar leaf, nutmeg and pine oils. Coca Cola was originally marketed as a 'nerve tonic,' containing various essential oils of citrus and spices.

However, essential oils cannot be trademarked, patented or controlled, and big pharma has little interest in pursuing something without monetary benefit. They do copy, mimic or try to reproduce synthetic versions of some essential oils, like the aforementioned Vick's Vaporub. But working with pure essential oils? No.

As far as clinical studies, from the 1980s to 1990s, there were more and more exciting studies of essential oils and their effects on chronic, metabolic and hormonal diseases. Then in 2001, there was a sudden stop in research – Dr. Schnaubelt in his book "The Healing Intelligence of Essential Oils" (2011) says "It does not appear outlandish to suspect reservations on the part of corporate pharmacology about remedies that may be too cheap and too accessible." (16)

It is also possible the fallacy developed or existed that antibiotics were wiping out diseases for good, and new research or development wasn't needed? In any case, there was a slow-down of studies.

Yet, new discoveries were made in the later 20th century, such as helichrysum essential oil able to mediate tissue protective and regenerative quality by going after free radicals; common essential oils were shown as effective agents to prevent osteoporosis, by Muhlbauer, Lozano, Palacio, Reinli and Felix; Dr. Anne-Marie Giraud-Robert's long-term studies have shown various essential oils are effective in treatment of hepatitis B and C.

Inhibit HMG CoA Reductase is a key enzyme in humans and plants. Essential oils can inhibit this enzyme and the synthesis of cholesterol which in turn is relevant for the prevention or the inhibition of carcinogensis and tumor growth shows. (17) Research has demonstrated that tumor cells can be shut off by essential oils.

"The intimate connection of essential oils to the evolution of enzymes in our bodies is but one factor that demonstrates how essential oils have naturally, from time immemorial, interfaced with humans." says Dr. Schnaubelt in "The Healing Intelligence of Plants." (18)

Looking at the chain of history, Romans got their knowledge of essential oils from the Greeks, who had gotten their knowledge from the Egyptians, who had gotten it from Sumeria and Babylonia. Europeans of the 18th century learned of essential oils from the 17th, and they from the 16th and on back. There was a "death period" in the Dark Ages, but nevertheless, through trade, wars and travels, the knowledge found a way back from the east to the west, and has survived. Now today, we are re-discovering, learning and taking the knowledge to new applications and potential modalities.

As we have started to cite a few medical studies, let's move to the next chapter where we have aggregated a number of studies and tests.

CHAPTER 3

THE WOW FACTOR: CLINICAL RESEARCH & STUDIES OF ESSENTIAL OILS

When a distinguished but elderly scientist states that something is possible, he is almost certainly right. When he states that something is impossible, he is very probably wrong.
~Arthur C. Clarke (1962)

Attempt the end and never stand to doubt;
Nothing's so hard, but search will find it out.
~ Robert Herrick Esq. (1648)

As you have read in the history section, there have been amazing people through time who tested, used, shared information, studied, classified and/or wrote about essential oils, aromatic plants and herbal remedies, from Hippocrates and Dioscordes to Avicenna, from the authors of the clay tablets found in Babylon to "The Leech Book of Bald" (with a recipe that kills MRSA) and Culpepper's "The English

Physician" right up to Gattefossé and our modern authors.

As the Tisserand Institute cites, the first published in vitro research on essential oils as antimicrobial agents was done in the 1800s: thyme oil and eucalyptus oil used as surgical antiseptics.(1)

Today, PubMed alone has more than 14,000 papers for essential oils research (and growing!), and quite a few of them have profound findings of validity. (PubMed is a service of the US National Library of Medicine® that: Provides free access to MEDLINE®, the NLM® database of indexed citations and abstracts to medical, nursing, dental, veterinary, health care, and preclinical sciences journal articles.)

In addition to PubMed, there are many more internationally recognized medical journals and sites reporting and publishing research.

We sometimes hear that "not much research has been done on essential oils" especially as an excuse by the medical community as to why they are not used in medical practice. I paraphrase Dr.

Schnaubelt on this subject:

> *The antibacterial activity of essential oils has been studied continually since the 1880s. Their efficacy against many bacterial pathogens has been demonstrated in countless in vitro experiments...suggesting that essential oils either inhibit bacterial growth or kill them outright. Possibly a most comprehensive study was done in the 1970s by Paul Belaiche, written in French. "The language barrier has provided an excuse for many Anglophonic guardians of pharmacological orthodoxy to act as it these studies never happened."* (2)

Here is another angle on the same subject, written by Valeria Ann Worwood in The Fragrant Mind. It concerns a Nobel Laureate, B. S. Blumberg, who got his Nobel Prize for discovering the hepatitis B virus and developing the blood test to detect it. He presented clinical research which proved hepatitis B was eliminated from 59% of people treated for 30 days with a dried and powered Phyllanthus amarus – a plant used for more than 2000 year in Ayurveda, and also used in China, Nigeria, East and West Africa,

South America, the Caribbean and Central America.

She continues:

> *"Despite the fact that the plant is used so extensively, and the fact that it has now been studied for over 10 years and has shown no toxic or side effects in animals or humans, it will probably never reach the marketplace in Britain or America. Phyllanthus needs more than the keen advocacy of the eminent Blumberg... it needs tens of millions of dollars to go through clinical testing, and chemical companies aren't going to support that work because, to date, they have no intention of selling herbs."* (3)

And the situation of essential oils is similar as far as medical and pharmaceutical attention.

So, let's turn our attention to more modern medical and clinical work and research, and get a taste for what has happened and what is happening now.

Dr. Paul Valnet, MD (1920-1995) was one of the first modern medical doctors to research and write about the medical application of essential oils in modern times. His overall body of work and teaching, known to specialists around the world, earned him the name "father of modern phyto-aromatherapy".

As chief physician to the Joint Chiefs of Staff of the French armed forces, continued his research into essential oils and used phyto-aromatherapy to treat some of the country's most senior military figures. He also founded an aromatherapy school.

By the way, Dr. Valnet provided the inspiration for two schools of thought on aromatherapy: the so-called French school, which adopted a clinical and scientific approach, and the British school, which has taken a more specific path of holistic well-being.

Dr. Valnet was a visionary – he first raised concerns over "the dangers of an all-out reliance on chemicals, disastrous for the planet and for human health" in the 1950s. Since then, and more recently, there are abundant studies, research and clinical test on essential oils and medical applications.

Valnet and his colleagues discovered that essential oils were powerful oxygenators with the ability to act as carrying agents in the delivery of nutrients into the cells. For instance, they found in laboratory experiments that the essential oil from thyme literally destroys the anthrax bacillus, the typhoid bacillus, the glanders bacillus, staphylococcus, the diphtheria bacillus, the diphtheria bacillus, meningococcus, and Koch's bacillus (the bacteria responsible for tuberculous lesions.) (4,5)

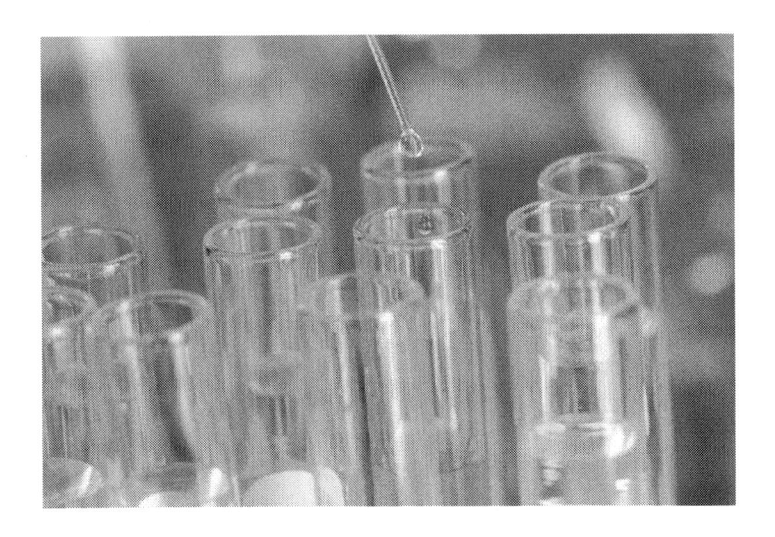

In the 1960s, classical studies were done by J.C. Maruzella and J. Pellecuer regarding essential oil efficiency against fungi and yeasts. Building on those studies in the 1990s, a study showed that the key enzyme in fungi was inhibited by essential oils.

Hildebert Wagner was a long-term professor of pharmaceutical biology at Munich's Ludwig Maximilian University. He published key studies on the spamolytic and sedative qualities of essential oils.

In the 1980s, classical studies were published showing the anti-inflammatory effects of chamomile, and that many essential oils with sesquiterpene components have anti-inflammatory effects.

This is a great study regarding airborne microbes and essential oils:

> French Professor Griffon, Director of the French Police Toxicology Laboratory, tested the antiseptic effect of a blend of essential oils that included Pine, Thyme, Peppermint, Lavender, Rosemary and Clove. He tested the ability of the EOs to purify the air of harmful disease-causing bacteria. Professor Griffon proceeded to set up a number of petri dishes about 6" off the floor and allowed them to collect microbes

for 24 hours. The dishes contained 210 colonies of various microbes, including numerous molds and staphylococci. Next, he sprayed an aerosol mixture of the essential oils into the air of the room. After only 15 minutes, only 14 colonies of microorganisms out of the original 210 were left alive. After 30 minutes, only four colonies of the original 210 were left. Within 30 minutes ALL of the potentially harmful, disease-causing molds and staphylococci were destroyed. (6)

Dr. Valnet also reported that in 1960, Dr. Bidadult's "clinical observations proved that the disinfection of the air surrounding the patient has therapeutic preventative effect." He used a mixture of pine, thyme, peppermint, lavender, rosemary, clove and cinnamon as a preventative for infectious childhood diseases such as whooping cough, coryza of nasal catarrh, influenza and acute or chronic diseases of the respiratory tract in adults (influenza, tuberculosis and pneumonia).

In 1985, a notable French researcher, Dr. Jean C. Lapraz, reported that he couldn't find a single bacteria or virus that could live in the presence of the essential oils of Cinnamon or Oregano. (7)

A Weber State University study proved conclusively that essential oils sprayed as a micro-fine mist into an enclosed atmosphere are more reliably effective than antibiotics such as Penicillin and Ampicillin. Viruses and bacteria will mutate to defend themselves against vaccines and antibiotics, but no pathogen has ever been known to mutate when confronted with essential oils. Essential Oils are far too complex, and their healing "code" cannot be cracked. (8)

As today's growing crisis of antibiotic-resistant bacteria, "super bugs", mutating viruses, infectious fungi and disease causing parasites are becoming more and more of a threat, essential oils may be able to resolve the issues, with study and proper use.

Prior to the mid 1980's, not many studies have been done about the effects on viruses, with more focus being given to bacterial studies. But in 1987, Lembke and Deininger published a ground-breaking study on antiviral properties of essential oils (they also included antibacterial and antifungal studies).

"The intimate connection of essential oils to the evolution of enzymes in our bodies is but one factor that demonstrates how essential oils have naturally, from time immemorial, interfaced with humans." (9)

A 1994 study at New York's Memorial Sloan-Kettering Cancer Center found that the vanilla-like aroma of heliotropin significantly reduced anxiety in patients undergoing MRI scans.(10)

In England in 2002, researchers found that applying lemon balm oil to the faces and arms of patients with severe dementia reduced their agitation by 35 percent. The study was published in the Journal of Clinical Psychiatry. (11)

At Wesleyan University in Connecticut, researchers found that the scent of lavender increased deep, restful sleep for both men and women (12); a Korean study published the same year (2006) came to the same conclusion (but the study only included women).

In 2009, researchers at the University of Leicester

examined AKBA or "acetyl-11-keto-beta-boswellic acid" and found positive benefits. This study was titled, "Frankincense Superior to Chemotherapy in Killing Late-Stage Ovarian Cancer Cells." (13) This is not the first study to suggest anti-cancer properties. The results of another study proved that frankincense oil could help with bladder cancer. The lead researcher Kamla Al-Salmani, a PhD student from the University's Department of Cancer Studies and Molecular Medicine explained:

"After a year of studying the AKBA compound with ovarian cancer cell lines in vitro, we have been able to show it is effective at killing the cancer cells. Frankincense is taken by many people with no known side effects. This finding has enormous potential to be taken to a clinical trial in the future and developed into an additional treatment for ovarian cancer." (14)

THERE ARE SO MANY THOUSANDS OF STUDIES, SO WE HAVE SIMPLY LISTED A SELECTION HERE TO GIVE YOU SOME BACKGROUND

Mark Barton Frank, Qing Yang, Jeanette Osban,

Joseph T Azzarello, Marcia R Saban, Ricardo Saban, Richard A Ashley, Jan C Welter, Kar-Ming Fung, Hsueh-Kung Lin. Department of Urology, University of Oklahoma Health Sciences Center, Oklahoma City, OK 73104, USA. frank@omrf.org Published Date: Dec 31, 2008
http://www.ncbi.nlm.nih.gov/pubmed/19296830

BACKGROUND: Originating from Africa, India, and the Middle East, frankincense oil has been important both socially and economically as an ingredient in incense and perfumes for thousands of years. Frankincense oil is prepared from aromatic hardened gum resins obtained by tapping Boswellia trees. One of the main components of frankincense oil is boswellic acid, a component known to have anti-neoplastic properties. The goal of this study was to evaluate frankincense oil for its anti-tumor activity and signaling pathways in bladder cancer cells.

CONCLUSION: Frankincense oil appears to distinguish cancerous from normal bladder cells and suppress cancer cell viability. Microarray and bioinformatics analysis proposed multiple pathways that can be activated by frankincense oil to induce bladder cancer cell death. Frankincense oil might represent an alternative intravesical agent for bladder cancer treatment.

Effects of aroma hand massage on pain, state anxiety and depression in hospice patients with terminal cancer. Department of Nursing, Keimyung University, Jung-gu, Daegu, Korea. Article Published Date: Jul 31, 2008. http://www.ncbi.nlm.nih.gov/pubmed/18753801

PURPOSE: The purpose of this study was to examine the effects of aroma hand massage on pain, state anxiety and depression in hospice patients with terminal cancer.

RESULTS: The aroma hand massage experimental group showed more significant differences in the changes of pain score (t=-3.52, p=.001) and depression (t=-8.99, p=.000) than the control group.

CONCLUSION: Aroma hand massage had a positive effect on pain and depression in hospice patients with terminal cancer.

ABSTRACT From the *Department of Anesthesia, Carolinas Medical Center University, Charlotte, NC

BACKGROUND: Postoperative nausea (PON) is a common complication of anesthesia and surgery. Antiemetic medication for higher-risk patients may reduce but does not reliably prevent PON. We examined aromatherapy as a treatment for patients experiencing PON after ambulatory surgery. Our primary hypothesis was that in comparison with inhaling a placebo, PON will be reduced significantly by aromatherapy with (1) essential oil of ginger, (2) a blend of essential oils of ginger, spearmint, peppermint, and cardamom, or (3) isopropyl alcohol. Our secondary hypothesis was that the effectiveness of aromatherapy will depend upon the agent used.
RESULTS: A total of 1151 subjects were screened for inclusion; 303 subjects reporting nausea were enrolled (26.3%), and 301 meeting protocol were analyzed (26.2%). The change in nausea level was significant for the blend ($P < 0.001$) and ginger ($P = 0.002$) versus saline but not for alcohol ($P < 0.76$).

The number of antiemetic medications requested after aromatherapy was also significantly reduced with ginger or blend aromatherapy versus saline ($P = 0.002$ and $P < 0.001$, respectively).

CONCLUSION: The hypothesis that aromatherapy would be effective as a treatment for PON was supported. On the basis of our results, future research further evaluating aromatherapy is warranted. Aromatherapy is promising as an inexpensive, noninvasive treatment for PON that can be administered and controlled by patients as needed.

A SAMPLING LIST OF CLINICAL RESEARCH AND STUDIES WITH ESSENTIAL OILS

S. Akhondzadeh, L. Kashani, A. Fotouhi et al., "Comparison of Lavandula angustifolia Mill. tincture and imipramine in the treatment of mild to moderate depression: a double-blind, randomized trial," Progress in Neuro-Psychopharmacology and Biological Psychiatry, vol. 27, no. 1, pp. 123–127, 2003.

Al-Hader, A.A., Hasan, Z.A., Aqel, M.B. (1994). Hyperglycemic and insulin release inhibitory effects of rosmarinus officinalis. Journal of Ethnopharmacology, 43, 217,22.

R. Alnamer, K. Alaoui, H. Bouidida el, et al., "Sedative and hypnotic activities of the methanolic and aqueous extracts of Lavandula officinalis from Morocco," Advances in Pharmacological Sciences, vol. 2012, Article ID 270824, 5 pages, 2012.

Al-Shuneigat, J., Cox, S. D., & Markham, J. L. (2005). Effects of a topical essential oil-containing formulation on biofilm-forming coagulase-negative staphylococci. Letters in Applied Microbiology, 41(1), 52-55.

D. T. Altaei, "Topical lavender oil for the treatment of recurrent aphthous ulceration," American Journal of Dentistry, vol. 25, no. 1, pp. 39–43, 2012.

Anderson, L., Gross, J. (2004). Aromatherapy with peppermint, isopropyl alcohol, or placebo is equally effective in relieving postoperative nausea. Journal of Peri-Anesthesia Nursing, 19(1), 29-35.

S. Atanossova-Shopova and K. S. Roussinov, "On certain central neurolotropic effects of lavender essential oil," Bulletin of the Institute of Physiology, vol. 8, pp. 69–76, 1970.

Atsumi T, Tonosaki K. Smelling lavender and rosemary increases free radical scavenging activity and decreases cortisol level in saliva. Psychiatry Res. 2007;150(1):89-96.

Bagetta G, Morrone LA, Rombola L, et al. Neuropharmacology of the essential oil of bergamot. Fitoterapia. 2010;81(6):453-61.

Bagg, J., Jackson, M. S., Petrina Sweeney, M., Ramage, G., & Davies, A. N. (2006). Susceptibility to melaleuca alternifolia (tea tree) oil of yeasts isolated from the mouths of patients with advanced cancer. Oral Oncology, 42(5), 487-492.

Ballard, C.G., O'Brien, J.T., Reichelt, K., Perry, E.K. (2002). Aromatherapy as a safe and effective treatment for the management of agitation in severe dementia: the results of a double-blind, placebo-controlled trial with Melissa. Journal of Clinical Psychiatry, 63, 553-8.

Barker, S & Altman P. (2010). A randomized, assessor blind, parallel group comparative efficacy trial of three products for the treatment of head lice in children – melaleuca oil and lavender oil, pyrethrins and piperonyl butoxide, and a “suffocation” product. BMC Dermatology, 10, 6.

Bassett, I. B., Pannowitz, D. L., & Barnetson, R. S. (1990). A comparative study of tea-tree oil versus benzoylperoxide in the treatment of acne. Med J Aust, 153(8), 455-458.

Bastard J, Tiran D. Aromatherapy and massage for antenatal anxiety: its effect on the fetus.Complement Ther Clin Pract. 2006;12(1):48-54.

Benencia, F. (1999). Antiviral activity of sandalwood oil against Herpes simplex viruses-1 and -2. Phytomedicine, 6(2), 119-23.

Bernardes W, Lucarini R, Tozatti M, Flauzino L, Souza

M, Turatti I, Andrade e Silva M, martins C, da Silva Filho A & Cunha W. (2010). Antibacterial activity of the essential oil from Rosmarinus officinalis and its major components against oral pathogens. Journal of Biosciences; 65(9-10):588-93.

Blackburn L, Achor S, Allen B, Bauchmire N, Dunnington D, Klisovic RB, Naber SJ, Roblee K, Samczak A, Tomlinson-Pinkham K, Chipps E. (2017). The Effect of Aromatherapy on Insomnia and Other Common Symptoms Among Patients With Acute Leukemia. Oncol Nurs Forum. 2017 Jul 1.

Bouhdid, S, Abrini, J, Zhiri, A, Espuny, M & Manresa, A. (2009). Investigation of functional and morphological changes in Pseudomonas aeruginosa and Staphylococcus aureus cells induced by Origanum compactum essential oil. Journal of Applied Microbiology, 106(5), 1558-1568.

Brady, A., Loughlin, R., Gilpin, D., Kearney, P., & Tunney, M. (2006). In vitro activity of tea-tree oil against clinical skin isolates of meticillin-resistant and -sensitive staphylococcus aureus and coagulase-negative staphylococci growing planktonically and as biofilms. Journal of Medical Microbiology, 55(Pt 10), 1375-1380.

R. Braden, S. Reichow, and M. A. Halm, "The use of the essential oil Lavandin to reduce preoperative anxiety in surgical patients," Journal of Perianesthesia Nursing, vol. 24, no. 6, pp. 348–355, 2009.

B. F. Bradley, S. L. Brown, S. Chu, and R. W. Lea, "Effects of orally administered lavender essential oil on responses to anxiety-provoking film clips," Human Psychopharmacology, vol. 24, no. 4, pp. 319–330, 2009.

Brandao, F. M. (1986). Occupational allergy to lavender oil. Contact Dermatitis, Vol 15, no 4, pgs 249-50.

G. Buchbauer, L. Jirovetz, W. Jäger, H. Dietrich, and C. Plank, "Aromatherapy: evidence for sedative effects of the essential oil of lavender after inhalation," Zeitschrift fur Naturforschung, vol. 46, no. 11-12, pp. 1067–1072, 1991

Buckle, J. (2007). Literature review: should nursing take aromatherapy more seriously? British Journal of Nursing, 16(2), 116-120.

Burns, E., Blamey, C., Ersser, S. J., Barnetson, L., & Lloyd, A. (2000). An investigation into the use of aromatherapy in intrapartum midwifery Practice. The Journal of Alternative and Complementary Medicine, 6(2), 141-7.

Burns, E., Zobbi, V., Panzeri, D., Oskrochi, R., Regalia, A. (2007). Aromatherapy in childbirth: a pilot randomized controlled trial. BJOG: An International Journal of Obstetrics & Gynaecology, 114(7), 838-44.

Burt, S. A. (2003). Antibacterial activity of selected plant essential oils against Escherichia coli O157:H7. Letters in Applied Microbiology 36, 162-7.

Burt, S. "Essential oils: their antibacterial properties and potential applications in foods--a review." Int J Food Microbiol. 2004 Aug 1;94(3):223-53.

Büyükokuroğlu, A. Gepdiremen, A. Hacimüftüoğlu, and M. Oktay, "The effects of aqueous extract of Lavandula angustifolia flowers in glutamate-induced neurotoxicity of cerebellar granular cell culture of rat pups," Journal of Ethnopharmacology, vol. 84, pp. 91–94, 2003

Caelli, M., Porteous, J., Carlson, C. F., Heller, R., & Riley, T. V. (2001). Tea tree oil as an alternative topical decolonization agent for methicillin-resistant Staphylococcus Aureus. The International Journal of Aromatherapy, 11(2). [Originally published in The Journal of Hospital Infection (2000), 46, 236-237.]

Canyon, D & Speare, R. (2007). A comparison of botanical and synthetic substances commonly used to prevent health lice (Pediculus humanus var. capitis) infestation. International Journal of Dermatology, 46(4), 422-426.

Cappello, G, Spezzaferro, M, Grossi, L, et al. (2007). Peppermint oil (Mintoil) in the treatment of irritable bowel syndrome: A prospective double blind placebo-controlled randomized trial. Digestive & Liver Disease,

39(6), 530-536.

Carson, C. F., Hammer, K. A., & Riley, T. V. (2006). Melaleuca alternifolia (tea tree) oil: A review of antimicrobial and other medicinal properties. Clinical Microbiology Reviews, 19(1), 50-62.
H. M. A. Cavanagh and J. M. Wilkinson, "Biological activities of lavender essential oil," Phytotherapy Research, vol. 16, no. 4, pp. 301–308, 2002.

Cermelli, C., Fabio, A., Fabio, G. and Quaglio, P. (2008) Effect of eucalyptus essential oil on respiratory bacteria and viruses. Current Microbiology 56, 1, 89-92.

Chang SY (2008) Effects of aroma hand massage on pain, state anxiety and depression in hospice patients with terminal cancer. Taehan Kanho Hakhoe Chi 38: 493-502 (Article in Korean). Cited by Dobetsberger C, Buchbauer G (2011) Actions of essential oils on the central nervous system: an updated review. Flavour and Fragrance Journal 26 (5): 300

L. W. Chien, S. L. Cheng, and C. F. Liu, "The effect of

lavender aromatherapy on autonomic nervous system in midlife women with insomnia," Evidence-Based Complementary and Alternative Medicine, vol. 2012, Article ID 740813, 8 pages, 2012.

M. Ching, "Contemporary therapy: aromatherapy in the management of acute pain?" Contemporary Nurse, vol. 8, no. 4, pp. 146–151, 1999.

Chung, M, Cho, S, Bhuiyan, M, Kim, K & Lee, S. (2010). Anti-diabetic effects of lemon balm (Melissa officinalis) essential oil on glucose- and lipid-regulating enzymes in type 2 diabetic mice. British J of Nutrition, 104(2), 180-188.

P. Conrad and C. Adams, "The effects of clinical aromatherapy for anxiety and depression in the high risk postpartum woman—a pilot study," Complementary Therapies in Clinical Practice, vol. 18, no. 3, pp. 164–168, 2012. View at Publisher • View at Google Scholar

Cooke, B., Ernst, E. (2000). Review: aromatherapy massage is associated with small, transient reductions in anxiety. British Journal of General Practice, 50, 493-6.

A. Dale and S. Cornwell, “The role of lavender oil in relieving perineal discomfort following childbirth: a blind randomized clinical trial,” Journal of Advanced Nursing, vol. 19, no. 1, pp. 89–96, 1994.

Daniel, A.N., Sartoretto, S.M., Schmidt, G., Caparroz-Assef, M., Bersani-Amado, C.A. and Cuman, R.K.N. (2008) Antiinflammatory and antinociceptive activities of eugenol essential oil in experimental animal models. Brazilian Journal of Pharmacognosy 19, 212-217.

Davies, SJ, Harding, LM & Baranowski, AP. (2002). A novel treatment of postherpetic neuralgia using peppermint oil. Clinical Journal of Pain, 18(3), 200-2.

J. Degel and E. P. Köster, “Odors: implicit memory and performance effects,” Chemical Senses, vol. 24, no. 3, pp. 317–325, 1999.

De Groot, A.C., & Weyland, W. (1992). Systemic

contact dermatitis from tea tree oil. Contact Dermatitis, 27, 279-80.

S. S. Denner, "Lavandula angustifolia miller: English lavender," Holistic Nursing Practice, vol. 23, no. 1, pp. 57–64, 2009

de Oliveira MM, Brugnera DF, Piccoli RH. "Essential oils of thyme and Rosemary in the control of Listeria monocytogenes in raw beef." Braz J Microbiol. 2014 Mar 10;44(4):1181-8. eCollection 2013.

M. A. Diego, N. A. Jones, T. Field et al., "Aromatherapy positively affects mood, EEG patterns of alertness and math computations," International Journal of Neuroscience, vol. 96, no. 3-4, pp. 217–224, 1998.

Dryden, M., Dailly, S., Crouch, M. (2004). A randomized, controlled trial of tea tree topical preparations versus a standard topical regimen for thc clearance of MRSA colonization. Journal of Hospital Infec, 56(4), 283-6.

C. Dunn, J. Sleep, and D. Collett, "Sensing an improvement: an experimental study to evaluate the use of aromatherapy, massage and periods of rest in an intensive care unit," Journal of advanced nursing, vol. 21, no. 1, pp. 34–40, 1995.

Dunning T. Applying a quality use of medicines framework to using essential oils in nursing practice. Complement Ther Clin Pract. 2005;11(3):172-81.

Dwivedi, C. & Zhang, Y. (1999). Sandalwood oil prevents skin tumour development in CD1 mice. European Journal of Cancer Prevention, 8, 449-55.

Edris AE. Pharmaceutical and therapeutic potentials of essential oils and their individual volatile constituents: a review. Phytother Res. 2007;21(4):308-23.

Edwards-Jones, V., Buck, R., Shawcross S.G., Dawson, M.M. and Dunn, K. (2004) The effect of essential oils on methicillin-resistant Staphylococcus aureus using a dressing model. Burns 30, 8, 772-777.

El Khoury, R., Atoui A., Mathieu F, Kawtharani H, El Khoury A, Maroun RG. Antifungal and Antiochratoxigenic Activities of Essential Oils and Total Phenolic Extracts: A Comparative Study. Antioxidants (Basel, Switzerland). 2017 Jul 9.

E. Elisabetsky, L. F. S. Brum, and D. O. Souza, "Anticonvulsant properties of linalool in glutamate-related seizure models," Phytomedicine, vol. 6, no. 2, pp. 107–113, 1999. Edris, A. (2007). Pharmaceutical and therapeutic potentials of essential oils and their individual volatile constituents: A review. Phytotherapy Research, 21, 308-323.

Enshaieh, S., Jooya, A., Siadat, A. H., & Iraji, F. (2007). The efficacy of 5% topical tea tree oil gel in mild to moderate acne vulgaris: A randomized, double-blind placebo-controlled study. Indian Journal of Dermatology, Venereology & Leprology, 73(1), 22-25.

Fadli M, Saad A, Sayadi S, Chevalier J, Mezrioui NE, Pagès JM, Hassani L. "Antibacterial activity of Thymus maroccanus and Thymus broussonetii essential oils against nosocomial infection - bacteria and their synergistic potential with antibiotics." Phytomedicine. 2012 Mar 15;19(5):464-71. doi: 10.1016/j.phymed.2011.12.003.

Fellowes D, Barnes K, Wilkinson S. Aromatherapy and massage for symptom relief in patients with cancer. Cochrane Database Syst Rev. 2004;(2):CD002287.

Fowler NA. Aromatherapy, used as an integrative tool for crisis management by adolescents in a residential treatment center. J Child Adolesc Psychiatr Nurs. 2006;19(2):69-76.

Fu, Y.-J., Zu, Y.-G., Chen, L.-Y., Shi, X.-G., Wang, Z., Sun, S. and Efferth, T. (2007) Antimicrobial activity of clove and rosemary essential oils alone and in combination. Phytotherapy Research 21, 989-994.

Furneri, P. M., Paolino, D., Saija, A., Marino, A., & Bisignano, G. (2006). In vitro antimycoplasmal activity of melaleuca alternifolia essential oil. Journal of Antimicrobial Chemotherapy, 58(3), 706-707.

Gao, Y. Y., Di Pascuale, M. A., Li, W., Baradaran-Rafii, A., Elizondo, A., Kuo, C. L., et al. (2005). In vitro and in vivo killing of ocular demodex by tea tree oil. British Journal of Ophthalmology, 89(11), 1468-1473.

Garozzo A, Timpanarao R, Stivala A, Bisignano G & Castro A. (2010) Activity of Melaleuca alternifolia (tea tree) oil on influenza virus A/PR/8: Study on the mechanism of action. Antiviral Research, 89(1), 83-8.

Gedney, J., Glover, T., Fillingim, R. (2004). Sensory and affective pain discrimination after inhalation of essential oils. Psychosomatic Medicine, 66(4), 599-606.

A. H. Gilani, N. Aziz, M. A. Khan et al., "Ethnopharmacological evaluation of the anticonvulsant, sedative and antispasmodic activities of Lavandula stoechas L," Journal of Ethnopharmacology, vol. 71, no. 1-2, pp. 161–167, 2000.

Gobel, H., Schmidt, G. and Soyka, D. (1994) Effect of

peppermint and eucalyptus oil preparations on neurophysiological and experimental algesimetric headache parameters. Cephalagia 14, 228-234

A. Gorji, "Pharmacological treatment of headache using traditional persian medicine," Trends in Pharmacological Sciences, vol. 24, no. 7, pp. 331–334, 2003.

Greenway, f, Frome & Engels, T. (2003). Temporary relief of postherpetic neuralgia pain with topical geranium oil. American J of Medicine, 115, 586-587.

Guimarães, A.G., Quintans, J.S.S. and Quintans-Júnior, L.J. (2013) Monoterpenes with analgesic activity – a systematic review. Phytotherapy Research 27, 1-15.

J. Guillmain, A. Rousseau, and P. Delaveau, "Effets neurodepresseurs de l'huile essentielle de lavandula augustifolia Mill," Annales Pharmaceutiques, vol. 47, pp. 337–343, 1989.

Gustafson, J. E., Chew, S., Markham, J., Bell, H.C.,

Wyllie, S. G., & Warmington, J. R. (1988). Effects of tea tree oil on Escherichia coli. Letters in Applied Microbiology, 26, 194-8.

Hadfield, N. (2001). The role of aromatherapy massage in reducing anxiety in patients with malignant brain tumors. International Journal of Palliative Nursing, 7(6), 279-285.

N. Hadi and A. A. Hanid, “Lavender essence for post-cesarean pain,” Pakistan Journal of Biological Sciences, vol. 14, no. 11, pp. 664–667, 2011.

Hajhashemi, V., Ghannadi, A., & Sharif, B. (2003). Anti-inflammatory and analgesic properties of the leaf extracts and essential oil of lavandula angustifolia mill. Journal of Ethnopharmacology, 89(1), 67-71.

Halm, M. (2008). Essential oils for management of symptoms in critically ill patients. American Journal of Critical Care, 17(2), 160-163.

Hammer, K. A., & Riley, T. V. (1998). In-vitro activity of essential oils, in particular Melaleuca alternifolia (tea tree) oil and tea tree oil products, against Candida spp. Journal of Antimicrobial Chemotherapy, 42, 591-5.

Hammer, K. A., Carson, C. F., & Riley, T. V. (2004). Antifungal effects of melaleuca alternifolia (tea tree) oil and its components on candida albicans, candida glabrata and saccharomyces cerevisiae. Journal of Antimicrobial Chemotherapy, 53(6), 1081-1085.

Hammer, K. A., Carson, C. F., Riley, T. V., & Nielsen, J. B. (2006). A review of the toxicity of Melaleuca alternifolia (tea tree) oil. Food & Chemical Toxicology, 44(5), 616-625.

Hammer K. A, & Carson C (2011) Antibacterial and antifungal activities of essential oils. In: Thormar, H. (ed) Lipids and Essential Oils as Antimicrobial Agents. Wiley, Chichester.

Han, S., Hur M., Buckle, J., Choi, J., Lee, M. (2006). Effect of aromatherapy on symptoms of dysmenorrheal in college students: A randomized placebo-controlled clinical trial. The Journal of

Alternative and Complentary Medicine, 12(6), 535-41.

Hansen, T., Hansen, B., Ringdal, G. (2006). Does aromatherapy massage reduce job-related stress? Results from a randomized, controlled trial. International Journal of Aromatherapy, 16(2), 89-94.

D. Hartman and J. C. Coetzee, "Two US practitioners' experience of using essential oils for wound care," Journal of Wound Care, vol. 11, no. 8, pp. 317–320, 2002.

Hayashi, K., & Hayashi, T. (1994). Virucidal effects of the steam distilate from Houttuynia cordata and its components on HSV-1, influenza virus, and HIV. Planta Medica, 61, 237-41.

Haze, S, Sakai, K & Gozu, Y. (2002). Effects of fragrance inhalation on sympathetic activity in normal adults. Japanese Journal of Pharmacology, 90, 247-253.

Henley, D., Lipson, N., Korach, K., Bloch, C. (2007). Prepubertal gynecomastia linked to lavender and tea tree oils. The New England Journal of Medicine, 356(5), 479-485.

Herz RS. Aromatherapy facts and fictions: a scientific analysis of olfactory effects on mood, physiology and behavior. Int J Neurosci. 2009;119(2):263-90. Review.

K. Hirokawa, T. Nishimoto, and T. Taniguchi, "Effects of lavender aroma on sleep quality in healthy Japanese students," Perceptual & Motor Skills, vol. 114, no. 1, pp. 111–122, 2012.

C. Holmes, V. Hopkins, C. Hensford, V. MacLaughlin, D. Wilkinson, and H. Rosenvinge, "Lavender oil as a treatment for agitated behaviour in severe dementia: a placebo controlled study," International Journal of Geriatric Psychiatry, vol. 17, no. 4, pp. 305–308, 2002.

Hongratanaworakit, T. and Buchbauer, G. (2004) Evaluation of the harmonizing effect of ylang ylang on humans after inhalation. Planta Medica 70, 7, 632-636.

Hongratanaworakit, T. and Buchbauer, G. (2006) Relaxing effect of ylang ylang on humans after transdermal absorption. Phytotherapy Research 20, 9, 758-763.

L. Hritcu, O. Cioanca, and M. Hancianu, "Effects of lavender oil inhalation on improving scopolamine-induced spatial memory impairment in laboratory rats," Phytomedicine, vol. 19, no. 6, pp. 529–534, 2012.

Hu PH, Peng YC, Lin YT, Chang CS, Ou MC. Aromatherapy for reducing colonoscopy related procedural anxiety and physiological paramters: a randomized controlled study. Hepatogastroenterology. 2010;57(102-102):1082-6.

M. Y. Huang, M. H. Liao, Y. K. Wang, et al., "Effect of lavender essential oil on LPS-stimulated inflammation," American Journal of Chinese Medicine, vol. 40, no. 4, pp. 845–859, 2012.

R. Hudson, "The value of lavender for rest and activity in the elderly patient," Complementary Therapies in

Medicine, vol. 4, no. 1, pp. 52–57, 1996.

M. H. Hur, Y. S. Yang, and M. S. Lee, "Aromatherapy massage affects menopausal symptoms in Korean climacteric women: a pilot-controlled clinical trial," Evidence-Based Complementary and Alternative Medicine, vol. 5, no. 3, pp. 325–328, 2008.

Hwang JH (2006) The effects of the inhalation method using essential oils on blood pressure and stress responses of clients with essential hypertension. Taehan Kanhoe Hakhoe Chi 36 (7): 1123-1134. (Article in Korean)

Jiro Imanishi, Hiroko Kuriyama, Ichiro Shigemori, Satoko Watanabe, Yuka Aihara, Masakazu Kita, Kiyoshi Sawai, Hiroo Nakajima, Noriko Yoshida, Masahiro Kunisawa, Masanori Kawase, and Kenji Fukui. Anxiolytic Effect of Aromatherapy Massage in Patients with Breast Cancer. Evidence-Based Complementary and Alternative Medicine
Volume 6 (2009), Issue 1, Pages 123-128

Inouye, S., Yamaguchi, H. (2001). Antibacterial

activity of essential oils and their major constituents against respiratory tract pathogens by gaseous contact. Journal of Antimicrobial Chemotherapy, 47, 565-73.

Itai, T., Amayasu, H., Kuribayashi, M., Kawamura, N., Okada, M., Momose, A., Tateyama, T., Narumi, K., Waka, Kaneko, U.S. (2000). Psychological effects of aromatherapy on chronic hemodialysis patients. Psychiatry and Clinical Neurosciences, 54, 393-7.

Jandourek, A. & Vazquez, J. (1998). Efficacy of melaleuca oral solution for the treatment of fluconazole refractory oral candidiasis in AIDS patients. AIDS, 12, 1033-7.

D. Jimbo, Y. Kimura, M. Taniguchi, M. Inoue, and K. Urakami, “Effect of aromatherapy on patients with Alzheimer's disease,” Psychogeriatrics, vol. 9, no. 4, pp. 173–179, 2009.

Kane, FM, Brodie, EE, Couli, A, et al. (2004). The analgesic effect of odour and music upon dressing change. British Journal of Nursing, 13(19), S4-12.

Karsha PV, Lakshmi OB (2010) Antibacterial activity of black pepper (Piper nigrum Linn.) with special reference to its mode of action on bacteria. Indian Journal of Natural Products and Resources 1 (2): 213-215

Kejova K, Jorova D, Bendova H, Gajdos P & Kolarova H. (2010). Phototoxicity of essential oils intended for cosmetic use. Toxicology in Vitro, 24(8), 2084-9.

Khan, M, Zahin & Hassan, S. (2009). Inhibition of quorum sensing regulated bacterial functions by plant essential oils with special reference to clove oil. Letters in Applied Microbiology, 49, 354-360.

Y. Kim, M. Kim, H. Kim, and K. Kim, "Effect of lavender oil on motor function and dopamine receptor expression in the olfactory bulb of mice," Journal of Ethnopharmacology, vol. 125, no. 1, pp. 31–35, 2009.

Kim JT, Wajda M, Cuff G, et al., Evaluation of aromatherapy in treating postoperative pain: pilot study. Pain Pract. 2006;6(4):273-7.

H. M. Kim and S. H. Cho, "Lavender oil inhibits immediate-type allergic reaction in mice and rats," Journal of Pharmacy and Pharmacology, vol. 51, no. 2, pp. 221–226, 1999.

Kim, J. et al. (2006). Evaluation of aromatherapy in treating post-operative pain: pilot study. Pain Practice, 6(4), 273-277.

J. T. Kim, C. J. Ren, G. A. Fielding et al., "Treatment with lavender aromatherapy in the post-anesthesia care unit reduces opioid requirements of morbidly obese patients undergoing laparoscopic adjustable gastric banding," Obesity Surgery, vol. 17, no. 7, pp. 920–925, 2007.

Y. Kim, M. Kim, H. Kim, and K. Kim, "Effect of lavender oil on motor function and dopamine receptor expression in the olfactory bulb of mice," Journal of Ethnopharmacology, vol. 125, no. 1, pp. 31–35, 2009.

Kon, KV; Rai MK. "Plant essential oils and their constituents in coping with multidrug-resistant bacteria." Expert Rev Anti Infect Ther. 2012

Jul;10(7):775-90.

Krebs M. Promote wellness with aromatherapy. Adv Nurse Pract. 2006;14(5):41-4.

M. Kritsidima, T. Newton, and K. Asimakopoulou, "The effects of lavender scent on dental patient anxiety levels: a cluster randomised-controlled trial," Community Dentistry and Oral Epidemiology, vol. 38, no. 1, pp. 83–87, 2010.

Kuriyama H, Watanabe S, Nakaya T, et al., Immunological and Psychological Benefits of Aromatherapy Massage. Evid Based Complement Alternat Med. 2005;2(2):179-184.

Kyle G. Evaluating the effectiveness of aromatherapy in reducing levels of anxiety in palliative care patients: results of a pilot study. Complement Ther Clin Pract. 2006;12(2):148-55.

Langeveld WT, Veldhuizen EJ, Burt SA. "Synergy between essential oil components and antibiotics: a review." Crit Rev Microbiol. 2014 Feb;40(1):76-94

Lee CO. Clinical aromatherapy. Part II: Safe guidelines for integration into clinical practice. Clin J Oncol Nurs. 2003;7(5):597-8.

Lee IS, Lee GJ. [Effects of lavender aromatherapy on insomnia and depression in women college students]. Taehan Kanho Hakhoe Chi. 2006;36(1):136-43.

Lehrner, J., Marwinski, G., Lehr, S., Johren, P., & Deecke, L. (2005). Ambient odors of orange and lavender reduce anxiety and improve mood in a dental office. Physiology & Behavior, 86(1-2), 92-95.

Lemon, K. (2004). An assessment of treating depression and anxiety with aromatherapy. The International Journal of Aromatherapy, 14, 63-69.

G. T. Lewith, A. D. Godfrey, and P. Prescott, “A single-blinded, randomized pilot study evaluating the aroma of Lavandula augustifolia as a treatment for mild insomnia,” Journal of Alternative and Complementary Medicine, vol. 11, no. 4, pp. 631–637, 2005.

Li L, Lin ZG, Wang S, Su XL, Gong HR, Li HL, Hu FL, Zheng HQ. (2017) The effects of clove oil on the enzyme activity of Varroa destructor Anderson and Trueman (Arachnida: Acari: Varroidae). Saudi J Biol Sci. 2017 Jul.

Lin PW, Chan WC, Ng BF, Lam LC. Efficacy of aromatherapy (Lavandula angustifolia) as an intervention for agitated behaviours in Chinese older persons with dementia: a cross-over randomized trial. Int J Geriatr Psychiatry. 2007;22(5):405-10.

V. M. Linck, A. L. da Silva, M. Figueiró, E. B. Caramão, P. R. H. Moreno, and E. Elisabetsky, "Effects of inhaled Linalool in anxiety, social interaction and aggressive behavior in mice," Phytomedicine, vol. 17, no. 8-9, pp. 679–683, 2010.

M. Lis-Balchin and S. Hart, "Studies on the mode of action of the essential oil of lavender (Lavandula angustifolia P. Miller)," Phytotherapy Research, vol. 13, pp. 540–542, 1999.

López P, Sanchez C, Batlle R, Nerín C. "Vapor-phase

activities of cinnamon, thyme, and oregano essential oils and key constituents against foodborne microorganisms." J Agric Food Chem. 2007 May 30;55(11):4348-56.

Lucks, B.C., Sorensen, J., Veal, L. (2002). Vitex agnus-castus essential oil and menopausal balance: a self-care survey. Complementary Therapies in Nursing and Midwifery, 8, 148-54.

H. W. Ludvigson and T. R. Rottman, "Effects of ambient odors of lavender and cloves on cognition, memory, affect and mood," Chemical Senses, vol. 14, no. 4, pp. 525–536, 1989.

Maddocks-Jennings W, Wilkinson JM. Aromatherapy practice in nursing: literature review. J Adv Nurs. 2004;48(1):93-103.

S. Marchand and P. Arsenault, "Odors modulate pain perception: a gender-specific effect," Physiology & Behavior, vol. 76, no. 2, pp. 251–256, 2002.

R. Masago, T. Matsuda, Y. Kikuchi et al., "Effects of

inhalation of essential oils on EEG activity and sensory evaluation," Journal of Physiological Anthropology and Applied Human Science, vol. 19, no. 1, pp. 35–42, 2000.

McCaffrey R, Thomas DJ, Kinzelman AO. The effects of lavender and rosemary essential oils on test-taking anxiety among graduate nursing students. Holist Nurs Pract. 2009 Mar-Apr;23(2):88-93.

Mercier D, Knevitt A. Using topical aromatherapy for the management of fungating wounds in a palliative care unit. J Wound Care. 2005;14(10):497-8, 500-1.

Messager, S., Hammer, K. A., Carson, C. F., & Riley, T. V. (2005). Assessment of the antibacterial activity of tea tree oil using the european EN 1276 and EN 12054 standard suspension tests. Journal of Hospital Infection, 59(2), 113-125.

Mi-Yeon Cho, Eun Sil Min, Myung-Haeng Hur, and Myeong Soo Lee. Effects of Aromatherapy on the Anxiety, Vital Signs, and Sleep Quality of Percutaneous Coronary Intervention Patients in

Intensive Care Units. Evidence-Based Complementary and Alternative Medicine. Volume 2013 (2013), Article ID 381381, 6 pages

Millar, B & Moore, J. (2008). Successful topical treatment of hand warts in a paediatric patient with tea tree oil (Melaleuca alternifolia). Complementary Therapies in Clinical Practice, 14(4), 225-27.

M. Moeini, M. Khadibi, R. Bekhradi, et al., "Effect of aromatherapy on the quality of sleep in ischemic heart disease patients hospitalized in intensive care units of heart hospitals of the Isfahan University of Medical Sciences," Iranian Journal of Nursing and Midwifery Research, vol. 15, no. 4, pp. 234–239, 2010.

N. Morris, "The effects of lavender (Lavendula angustifolium) baths on psychological well-being: two exploratory randomized controls trials," Complementary Therapies in Medicine, vol. 10, no. 4, pp. 223–228, 2002.

Moss, M., Hewitt, S. and Moss, L. (2008) Modulation of cognitive performance and mood by aromas of peppermint and ylang ylang. International Journal of Neuroscience 118, 59-77.

M. Moss, J. Cook, K. Wesnes, and P. Duckett, "Aromas of rosemary and lavender essential oils differentially affect cognition and mood in healthy adults," International Journal of Neuroscience, vol. 113, no. 1, pp. 15–38, 2003.

Nguyen, Q., Paton C. (2008). The use of aromatherapy to treat behavioral problems in dementia. International Journal of Geriatric Psychiatry, 23, 337-346.

Nostro A, Bisignano G, Angela Cannatelli M, Crisafi G, Paola Germanò M, Alonzo V. Effects of Helichrysum italicum extract on growth and enzymatic activity of Staphylococcus aureus. 2001.

Oyedele, A. O., Gbolade, A. A., Sosan, M.B., Adewoyin, F. B., Soyelu, O.L., & Orafidiya, O. O. (2002). Formulation of an effective mosquito-repellent topical product from Lemongrass oil. Phytomedicine, 9, 259-62.

Ou MC, Lee YF, Li CC, Wu SK (2014) The effectiveness of essential oils for patients with neck pain: a randomized controlled study. Journal of Alternative and Complementary Medicine 20 (10): 771-779

M. C. Ou, T. F. Hsu, A. C. Lai, et al., "Pain relief assessment by aromatic essential oil massage on outpatients with primary dysmenorrhea: a randomized, double-blind clinical trial," Journal of Obstetrics and Gynaecology Research, vol. 38, no. 5, pp. 817–822, 2012.

Parrish, Nicole; Boire, A; Reidel, S. Essential Oils and Future Antibiotics: New Weapons against Emerging Superbugs? Dept of Pathology, Division of Microbiology at The Johns Hopkins University, Baltimore, MD. Published June 03, 2013 http://www.esciencecentral.org/journals/essential-oils-and-future-antibiotics-new-weapons-against-emerging-superbugs-2329-8731.1000105.php?aid=14230

Patricia M. Complementary therapies for children: aromatherapy. Paediatr Nurs. 2004;16(7):28-30.

Pauli, A., & Schilcher, H. (2004). Specific Selection of Essential Oil Compounds for Treatment of Children's Infection Diseases. Pharmaceuticals, 1, 1–30.

N. S. L. Perry, P. J. Houghton, A. Theobald, P. Jenner, and E. K. Perry, "In-vitro inhibition of human erythrocyte acetylcholinesterase by Salvia lavandulaefolia essential oil and constituent terpenes," Journal of Pharmacy and Pharmacology, vol. 52, no. 7, pp. 895–902, 2000.

R. Perry, R. Terry, L. K. Watson, and E. Ernst, "Is lavender an anxiolytic drug? A systematic review of randomised clinical trials," Phytomedicine, vol. 19, pp. 825–835, 2012.

Perry N, Perry E. Aromatherapy in the management of psychiatric disorders: clinical and neuropharmacological perspectives. CNS Drugs. 2006;20(4):257-80.

Pinto, E., Vale-Silva, L., Cavaleiro, C. and Salguero, L. (2009) Antifungal activity of the clove essential oil from Syzygium aromaticum on Candida, Aspergillus and dermatophyte species. Journal of Medical Microbiology 58, 11, 1454-1462.

Price, S. & Price, L. (2007). Aromatherapy for health professionals, 3rd Ed. Philadelphia: Churchill Livingstone Elsevier.

L. Price, "The genesis of essential oils," in Aromatherapy for Health Professionals, S. Price and L. Price, Eds., pp. 3–18, Churchill Livingstone/Elsevier, Edinburgh, Scotland, 4th edition, 2012.

S. Price and S. A. Oram, "Care of the elderly," in Aromatherapy for Health Professionals, pp. 261–272, Churchill Livingstone/Elsevier, Edinburgh, UK, 4th edition, 2012.

Radulović, N. S., Blagojević, P. D., Stojanović-Radić, Z. Z., & Stojanović, N. M. (2013). "Antimicrobial plant metabolites: structural diversity and mechanism of action" Current Medicinal Chemistry, 20; 932–52.

Rho KH, Han SH, Kim KS, Lee MS. 'Effects of aromatherapy massage on anxiety and self-esteem in Korean elderly women: a pilot study.' Int J Neurosci. 2006;116(12):1447-55.
Richards D. Effect of essential oil mouthwashes on plaque and gingivitis. Evid Based Dent. 2017 Jun 23.

Rose, J. E. & Behm, F. M. (1994). 'Inhalation of vapor from black pepper extract reduced smoking withdrawal symptoms.' Drug and Alcohol Dependence, 34, 225-9.

D. N. Rutledge and C. J. Jones, "Effects of topical essential oil on exercise volume after a 12-week exercise program for women with fibromyalgia: A pilot study," Journal of Alternative and Complementary Medicine, vol. 13, no. 10, pp. 1099–1106, 2007.

Saeki, Y. (2000). The effect of foot bath with or without the essential oil of lavender on the autonomic nervous system: A randomized trial. Complementary Therapies in Medicine, 8, 2-7.

Seow, Y. X., Yeo, C. R., Chung, H. L., & Yuk, H.-G. (2014). Plant essential oils as active antimicrobial agents. Critical Reviews in Food Science and Nutrition, 54 (February 2015), 625–644.

W. N. Setzer, "Essential oils and anxiolytic aromatherapy," Natural Product Communications, vol. 4, no. 9, pp. 1305–1316, 2009.

Saab AM, Gambari R, Sacchetti G, Guerrini A, Lampronti I, Tacchini M, El Samrani A, Medawar S, Makhlouf H, Tannoury M, Abboud J, Diab-Assaf M, Kijjoa A, Tundis R, Aoun J, Efferth T. Phytochemical and pharmacological properties of essential oils from Cedrus species. Nat Prod Res. 2017 Jul 3.

T. Sakurada, H. Kuwahata, S. Katsuyama et al., "Chapter 18 intraplantar injection of Bergamot essential oil into the mouse hindpaw. Effects on capsaicin-induced nociceptive behaviors," International Review of Neurobiology, vol. 85, pp. 237–248, 2009.

Saljoughian S, Roohinejad S, Bekhit AEA, Greiner R, Omidizadeh A, Nikmaram N, Mousavi Khaneghah A. The effects of food essential oils on cardiovascular diseases: A review. Crit Rev Food Sci Nutr. 2017 Feb 10.

C. Sanders, M. Diego, M. Fernandez, T. Field, M. Hernandez-Reif, and A. Roca, "EEG asymmetry responses to lavender and rosemary aromas in adults and infants," International Journal of Neuroscience, vol. 112, no. 11, pp. 1305–1320, 2002.

Sanguinetti M, Posteraro B, Romano L, Battaglia T, Lopizzo T, De Carolis E, Fadda G (2007). In vitro activity of Citrus bergamia (bergamot) oil against clinical isolates of dermatophytes. Journal of Antimicrobial Chemotherapy 59 (2): 305-308

P. Sasannejad, M. Saeedi, A. Shoeibi, et al., "Lavender essential oil in the treatment of migraine headache: a placebo-controlled clinical trial," European Journal of Neurology, vol. 67, no. 5, pp. 288–291, 2012.

W. Sayorwan, V. Siripornpanich, T. Piriyapunyaporn,

T. Hongratanaworakit, N. Kotchabhakdi, and N. Ruangrungsi, “The effects of lavender oil inhalation on emotional states, autonomic nervous system, and brain electrical activity,” Journal of the Medical Association of Thailand, vol. 95, pp. 598–606, 2012.

Serafino, A., Vallebona et al. Stimulatory effect of Eucalyptus essential oil on innate cell-mediated immune response. 2008. BMC Immunology.

Setzer WN. Essential oils and anxiolytic aromatherapy. Nat Prod Commun. 2009;4(9):1305-16.

Shaaban, H.A.E., El-Ghorab, A.H. and Shibamoto, T. (2012) Bioactivity of essential oils and their volatile aroma components: review. Journal of Essential Oil Research 24, 2, 203-212.

Silva, J., Abebe, W., Sousa, S.M., Duarte, V.G., Machado, M.I.L. and Matos, F.J.A. (2003) Analgesic and anti-inflammatory effects of essential oils of eucalyptus. Journal of Ethnopharmacology 89, 277-83.

Singh, G; Kapoor, IPS; Pandey, SK; Singh, UK; et al. (2002). "Studies on essential oils: Part 10; Antibacterial activity of volatile oils of some spices". Phytotherapy Research 16 (7): 680–2. doi:10.1002/ptr.951. PMID 12410554

Sharma S, Araujo M, Wu M, Qaqush J & Charles C. (2010). Superiority of an essential oil mouthrinse when compared with a 0.05% cetylpyridinium chloride containing mouthrinse: A six-month study. International Dental Journal, 60(3), 175-80.

F. Sheikhan, F. Jahdi, E. M. Khoei, et al., “Episiotomy pain relief: use of Lavender oil essence in primiparous Iranian women,” Complementary Therapies in Clinical Practice, vol. 18, no. 1, pp. 66–70, 2012.

J. Shen, A. Niijima, M. Tanida, Y. Horii, K. Maeda, and K. Nagai, “Olfactory stimulation with scent of lavender oil affects autonomic nerves, lipolysis and appetite in rats,” Neuroscience Letters, vol. 383, no. 1-2, pp. 188–193, 2005.

Sherry, E., Warnke, P. H. (2001). Percutaneous

treatment of chronic MRSA osteomyelitis with a novel plant-derived antiseptic. BMC Surgery, 1(1).

Snow L, Hovanec L & Brandt J. (2004). A controlled trial of aromatherapy for agitation in nursing home patients with dementia. J Alternative & Complementary Medicine, 10(3), 431-437.

Solarte A, Astorga RJ, Aguiar F, Galán-Relaño Á, Maldonado A, Huerta B. Foodborne Pathog Dis. 2017 Jul 6. Combination of Antimicrobials and Essential Oils as an Alternative for the Control of Salmonella enterica Multiresistant Strains Related to Foodborne Disease.

Solórzano-Santos, F., & Miranda-Novales, M. G. (2012). "Essential oils from aromatic herbs as antimicrobial agents." Current Opinion in Biotechnology, 23 (April 2009), 136–141.

Soukoulis, S., & Hirsch, R. (2004). The effects of a tea tree oil-containing gel on plaque and chronic gingivitis. Australian Dental Journal, 49(2), 78-83.

D. P. de Sousa, F. F. F. Nóbrega, C. C. M. P. Santos, and R. N. de Almeida, "Anticonvulsant activity of the linalool enantiomers and racemate: investigation of chiral influence," Natural Product Communications, vol. 5, no. 12, pp. 1847–1851, 2010.

Srivasta, K. C., Mustafa, T. (1992). Ginger (Zingiber officinale) in Rheumatism and Musculoskeletal Disorders. Medical Hypotheses, 39, 342-8.

Štefanidesová K, Škultéty Ľ, Sparagano OAE, Špitalská E. The repellent efficacy of eleven essential oils against adult Dermacentor reticulatus ticks. Tick Borne Dis. 2017 Jun 15.

Tabassum, N., & Vidyasagar, G. M. (2013). "Antifungal investigations on plant essential oils. A review." International Journal of Pharmacy and Pharmaceutical Sciences, 5, 19–28.

Takarada, R. et al. (2004). A comparison of the antibacterial efficacies of essential oils against oral pathogens. Oral Microbiology and Immunology, 19, 61-64.

Thorgrimsen L, Spector A, Wiles A, Orrell M. Aroma therapy for dementia. Cochrane Database Syst Rev. 2003;(3):CD003150.

Toloza A, Zygadlo J, Biurrun F, Rotman A & Picollo M. (2010). Bioactivity of Argentinean essential oils against permethrin-resistant head lice, Pediculus humanus capita. J of Insect Science, 10, 185.

Torres Salazar A, Hoheisel J, Youns M & Wink M. (2011). Anti-inflammatory and anti-cancer activities of essential oils and their biological constituents. International J of Clinical Pharmacology & Therapeutics, 49(1), 93-95.

Tragoolpua, Y. and Jaatisatienr, A. (2007) Anti-herpes simplex virus activities of Eugenia caryophyllus (Spreng.) Bullock & S. G. Harrison and essential oil, eugenol. Phytotherapy Research 21, 12, 1153-1158.

Tyagi A & Malik A. (2010). Liquid and vapour-phase antifungal activities of selected essential oils against Candida albicans: Microscopic observations and chemical characterization of Cymbopogon citratus. BMC Complementary & Alternative Medicine, 10, 65.

P. Tysoe, "The effect on staff of essential oil burners in extended care settings," International Journal of Nursing Practice, vol. 6, no. 2, pp. 110–112, 2000.

T. Umezu, "Behavioral effects of plant-derived essential oils in the Geller type conflict test in mice," Japanese Journal of Pharmacology, vol. 83, no. 2, pp. 150–153, 2000.

Umezu, K. Nagano, H. Ito, K. Kosakai, M. Sakaniwa, and M. Morita, "Anticonflict effects of lavender oil and identification of its active constituents," Pharmacology Biochemistry and Behavior, vol. 85, no. 4, pp. 713–721, 2006.

K. Vakilian, M. Atarha, R. Bekhradi, and R. Chaman, "Healing advantages of lavender essential oil during episiotomy recovery: a clinical trial," Complementary Therapies in Clinical Practice, vol. 17, no. 1, pp. 50–53, 2011

Van der Ploeg E, Eppingstall B & O'Connor D. (2010). The study protocol of a blinded randomized-controleed cross-over trial of lavender oil as a treatment of behavioural symptoms in dementia. BMC Geriatrics, 10, 49.

Van Vuuren S, Holl D. Antimicrobial natural product research: A review from a South African perspective for the years 2009-2016. J Ethnopharmacol. 2017 Jul 7.

C. Villemure, B. M. Slotnick, and M. C. Bushnell, "Effects of odors on pain perception: deciphering the roles of emotion and attention," Pain, vol. 106, no. 1-2, pp. 101–108, 2003.

D. Wang, X. Yuan, T. Liu, et al., "Neuroprotective activity of lavender oil on transient focal cerebral ischemia in mice," Molecules, vol. 17, no. 8, pp. 9803–9817, 2012.

Warnke, PH; Becker, ST; Podschun, R; Sivananthan, S; et al. (2009). "The battle against multi-resistant strains: Renaissance of antimicrobial essential oils as a promising force to fight hospital-acquired infections". Journal of Cranio-Maxillofacial Surgery 37 (7): 392–7. doi:10.1016/j.jcms.2009.03.017. PMID 19473851.

Warnke PH, Lott AJ, Sherry E, Wiltfang J, Podschun R. The ongoing battle against multi-resistant strains: in-vitro inhibition of hospital-acquired MRSA, VRE, Pseudomonas, ESBL E. coli and Klebsiella species in the presence of plant-derived antiseptic oils. J Craniomaxillofac Surg. 2013 Jun;41(4):321-6. doi: 10.1016/j.jcms.2012.10.012.

T. I. Williams, "Evaluating effects of aromatherapy massage on sleep in children with autism: a pilot study," Evidence-Based Complementary and Alternative Medicine, vol. 3, no. 3, pp. 373–377, 2006.

Woelk, H & Schlafke, S. (2009). A multi-center, double-blind, randomizsed study of the lavender oil preparation Silexan in comparison to Lorazepam for generalized anxiety disorder. Phytomedicine, 17, 94-99.

A. Woolfson and D. Hewitt, "Intensive aromacare,"

International Journal of Aromatherapy, vol. 4, no. 2, pp. 12–13, 1992.

Woronuk G., Z. Demissie, M. Rheault, and S. Mahmoud, "Biosynthesis and therapeutic properties of lavandula essential oil constituents," Planta Medica, vol. 77, no. 1, pp. 7–15, 2011.

F. Xu, K. Uebaba, H. Ogawa et al., "Pharmaco-physio-psychologic effect of ayurvedic oil-dripping treatment using an essential oil from Lavendula angustifolia," Journal of Alternative and Complementary Medicine, vol. 14, no. 8, pp. 947–956, 2008.

K. Yamada, Y. Mimaki, and Y. Sashida, "Anticonvulsive effects of inhaling lavender oil vapour," Biological and Pharmaceutical Bulletin, vol. 17, no. 2, pp. 359–360, 1994.

Yang, S.-A., Jeon, S.-K., Lee, E.-J., Shim, E.-H. and Lee, I.-S. (2010) Comparative study of the chemical composition and antioxidant activity of six essential oils and their components. Natural Products Research

24, 140-151.

Yap, Polly Soo Xi; Beow Chin Yiap; Hu Cai Ping; and Swee Hua Erin Lim. “Essential Oils, A New Horizon in Combating Bacterial Antibiotic Resistance”. Open Microbiol J. 2014; 8: 6–14. Published online 2014 Feb 7.

Yap, Polly Soo Xi, Lim SH, Hu CP, Yiap BC. “Combination of essential oils and antibiotics reduce antibiotic resistance in plasmid-conferred multidrug resistant bacteria.” Phytomedicine. 2013 Jun 15;20(8-9):710-3.

Y. B. Yip and S. H. M. Tse, “The effectiveness of relaxation acupoint stimulation and acupressure with aromatic lavender essential oil for non-specific low back pain in Hong Kong: a randomised controlled trial,” Complementary Therapies in Medicine, vol. 12, no. 1, pp. 28–37, 2004.

Y. B. Yip and S. H. M. Tse, “An experimental study on the effectiveness of acupressure with aromatic lavender essential oil for sub-acute, non-specific neck pain in Hong Kong," Complementary Therapies in Clinical Practice, vol. 12, no. 1, pp. 18–26, 2006.

Y. B. Yip and A. C. Y. Tam, "An experimental study on the effectiveness of massage with aromatic ginger and orange essential oil for moderate-to-severe knee pain among the elderly in Hong Kong," Complementary Therapies in Medicine, vol. 16, no. 3, pp. 131–138, 2008.

CHAPTER 4

THE CRISIS OF "SUPERBUGS", ANTIBIOTICS AND ESSENTIAL OILS

Medicinal plants "offer our best hope for confronting drug-resistant bacteria."
~James Duke, Ph.D., retired U.S.D.A. botanist

"The fact that essential oils can kill bacteria that are resistant to antibiotics is amazing in itself. The fact that they can sometimes reverse antibiotic resistance in bacteria is seemingly miraculous."
~Robert Tisserand, The Tisserand Institute

Let's talk "superbugs". Antibiotic-resistant bacteria, otherwise known as "superbugs" are on the rise and have now been declared one of the Center for Disease Control's (CDC) top public health concerns.

Over the last decade, almost every type of bacteria has become stronger and less responsive to antibiotic treatment.

“These are nightmare bacteria that present a triple threat,” said Thomas Frieden, former director of the CDC, in a USA Today interview. “They’re resistant to nearly all antibiotics. They have high mortality rates, killing half of people with serious infections. And they can spread their resistance to other bacteria.” (1)

Overuse or misuse of antibiotics and antibacterial products – plus high use of antibiotics in our food chain (specifically chicken and cows) - has contributed strongly to these “superbugs.”

These are viruses, fungi, and bacteria that are antibiotic resistant and they are creating massive problems in hospitals, clinics, nursing homes, and soon on a wider “location-scale” worldwide. Those who become ill or infected find that antibiotics don’t work at all or are less effective, or must take much higher doses to make any impact. This is of course dangerous and potentially disastrous.

In a report written in 2010 by Rustam Aminov (University of Aberdeen in the UK), it is noted that the annual additional cost of treating hospital-acquired infections from just six species of antibiotic-resistant bacteria was estimated to be at least $1.3 billion in

1992 dollars ($1.87 billion in 2006 dollars) – more than the annual spending on influenza. (2)

Drug-resistant microbes could cause more than 10 million deaths by the year 2050. (3)

Former U.K. Prime Minister David Cameron warns: “If we fail to act, we are looking at an almost unthinkable scenario where antibiotics no longer work and we are cast back into the dark ages of medicine where treatable infections and injuries will kill once again." He calls for action to tackle the growing threat of resistance to antibiotics. (4)

Antibiotic-resistant superbugs are "the biggest threat to patient safety in the hospital that we have," said Costi Sifri, an infectious disease physician and hospital epidemiologist at the University of Virginia Health System. "Unfortunately, it doesn't seem like anything is slowing their spread." (5)

THE THREAT OF MRSA

Methicillin-resistant Staphylococcus aureus or MRSA is also known as staph infection - this type of bacterial contamination can be fatal and directly leads to more than 10,000 deaths every year.

These bacteria fester on the skin and in the soft tissue of the nose. What begins as small pimple-like bumps – similar in appearance to a spider bite – can abscess to the point that they must be medically drained and treated.

It is the most common form of skin infection in the United States and leads to pneumonia, surgical complications, and blood/bone infections.

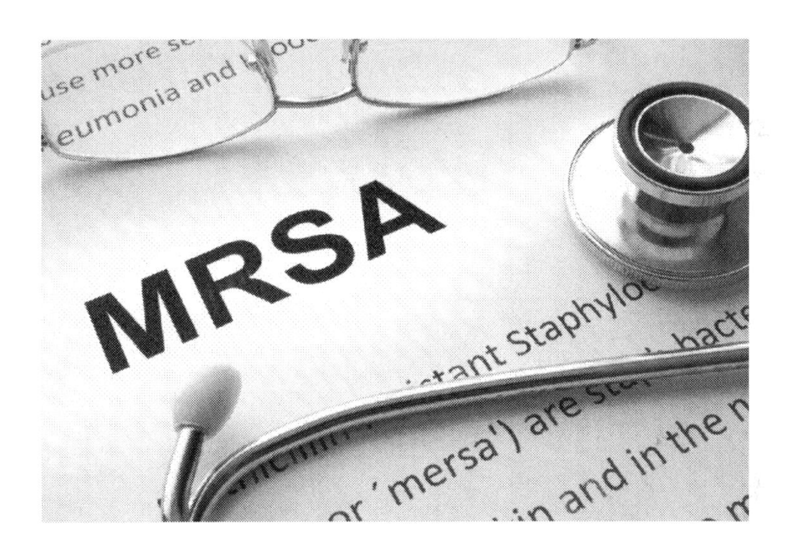

The majority of MRSA infections happen in the hospital among those who have weakened immune systems. They're called hospital-associated MRSA cases. However, those that happen outside a hospital environment are called community-associated MRSA and do occur.

CRE AND VRE EVEN A STRONGER THREAT

An even newer family of antibiotic-resistant bacteria than MRSA, known as CRE (Carbapenem-resistant Enterobacteriaceae) and vancomycin-resistant Enterococus (VRE), is raising concerns across the medical community because of the ability to cause infections that defy even the strongest antibiotics.

At this writing, CRE is currently only found in hospitals and nursing homes, unlike some of the other drug-resistant bacteria.

The antibiotic resistance is spread by mobile pieces of DNA that can move between different species of bacteria, creating new, drug-defying bugs. If this grows and spreads, common conditions affecting millions of Americans, which are now treated with antibiotics — such as diarrhea, urinary tract infections, respiratory conditions and pneumonia — could become untreatable. (6)

According to Cari Romm, a writer and researcher at The Atlantic, "in the U.S., antibiotic resistance caused more than two million illnesses in 2013, according to a report by the Centers for Disease Control and

Prevention, and an estimated 23,000 deaths," and they've also incurred an extra $20 billion in healthcare costs. (7)

Dr. Harold Neu, former Professor of Medicine at Columbia University, summarized: in 1941, only 40,000 units per day of penicillin for four days was required to cure pneumococcal pneumonia. "Today, a patient could receive 24 million units of penicillin a day and die of pneumococcal meningitis..." He concluded that bacteria are cleverer than men. (7B)

Dr. Richard Krause (deceased in 2015), the former senior scientific advisor at National Institutes of Health (NIH) said, "We forgot that microbes are restless and they would counterattack. That was incredible hubris on our part." (7C)

CAN ESSENTIAL OILS HELP SOLVE THIS PROBLEM?

YES.

According to James Duke, Ph.D., the retired U.S.D.A. botanist who studied herbs for many years, medicinal plants "offer our best hope for confronting drug-resistant bacteria." (8)

There is amazing research, clinic work and actual testing that shows essential oils not only can take on the issue but are doing so. Essential oils will probably evolve as the new weapon against the "superbugs" and emerge as a more natural way to fight bacterial and viruses.

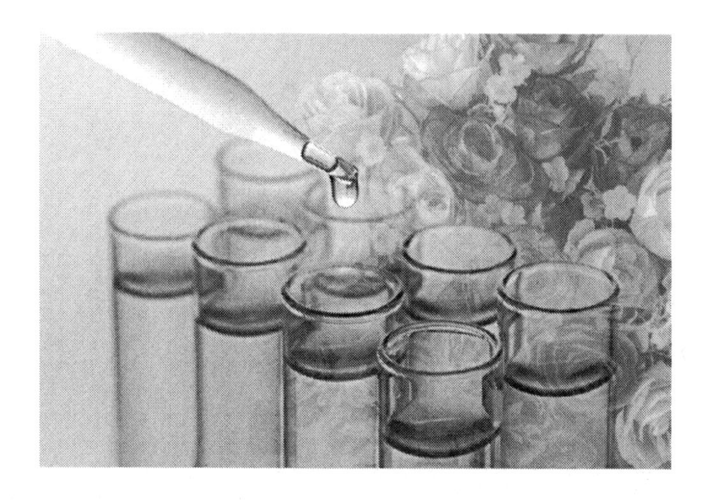

This is already happening informally among those in the know who use essential oils. And remember, a combination of essential oils beat the medieval Plague for the four thieves and others who survived. We know with certainty that most essential oils are anti-bacterial, anti-viral and anti-fungal. There is no question there are powers to be explored and applied to this current crisis.

In 2001 (in Australia at University of Sydney, Nepean Hospital), **we have the first (one of the few recorded in medical setting?) case MRSA being treated and beaten by essential oils** (a solution of eucalyptus and tea tree oils). A 49 year old man had a fracture of his left leg (had been run over by a golf cart). The fracture and soft tissues healed at 2 and 8 months later, but he needed more work. MRSA developed deep in the wound and bone, and amputation was considered, until Dr. Eugene Sherry took charge of the care and requested the essential oil treatment. At 3 months, his cultures were clear, the wound healed and symptoms resolved – and he kept his leg. (9A)

The paper by Dr. Sherry and his colleagues following the procedure ended with this summary: "A recent paper by Anderson and Fennessy (10) reviewed and concluded that there was compelling in vitro evidence of the effectiveness of tea tree oil against MRSA; here we add a clinical case." (10)

Another MRSA case was presented by Jimm Harrison at the Unlimited Possibilities, 8th Aromatherapy Conference on the Therapeutic Uses of

Essential Oils in 2015. A female patient in her mid 40s (with Type I diabetes) contracted MRSA following a foot wound. She was treated with a series of antiobiotics but they did not eradicate the infection. Amputation was the only option offered by the physician. The patient had sought alternatives - and began a series of IV's using a mix that included Cinnamon Bark (cinnamomum ceylanicum), chosen because of its strong antibacterial activity against MRSA. The IV's were complimented with injections to the affected area along with some topical preparations. The MRSA was reduced to **NO DETECTION OF BACTERIA** in the culture following 3 weeks of treatment. (9B)

These are two very encouraging and exciting cases!

Medical test trials were undertaken by a University of Sydney team, who discovered that the mixture of eucalyptus, tea tree, lemon, thyme, clove essential oil plus alcohol cured staphylococcus aureus, or "golden staph" infections, on two-thirds of hospital patients, where conventional antibiotics were ineffective.

Dr. Sherry said it isn't really a "new" discovery, because Australians have known about the healing powers of eucalyptus for a long time, and the Aborigines thousands of years before.

Essential oils have been eradicating diseases and microbes for centuries, just not formally recognized by the current medical or scientific world in the U.S. This might partly be because of the pharmaceutical lobby (we address that in Chapter 5), or a slower acceptance in the US by the medical world (we also address that in Chapter 5).

There are some tests and new awareness in U.S. scientific and medical circles coming to the forefront.

Dr. Andrew Weil says, following the release of an important Greek clinical study using essential oils on MRSA, "This is a return to the historical use of essential oils and welcome news. I hope that further research substantiates the findings. We need an effective way to counter MRSA, and if these results hold true, essential oils could be at least part of the solution. I have long recommended using a mixture of water plus lavender or tea tree essential oils for an environmentally and people-friendly antibacterial spray for kitchen or bathroom surfaces. In addition, studies have shown that a wash of one-percent basil essential oil effectively eliminates bacteria on fruits and vegetables, and is much friendlier to human beings and the environment than bleach." (11)

The study Dr. Weil references is covered later in this chapter. (12)

Researchers at Cornell University have found lavender oil can eradicate certain antibiotic-resistant bacteria, including more than one strain of pathogenic Staphylococcus and pathogenic Streptococcus often involved in coughs and colds. Edwards-Jones et al. (2004) found that a combination of Lavender, Geranium, and Tea Tree had an increased inhibitory effect on the growth of methicillin-resistant Staphylococcus aureus (MRSA), but that Lavender and Tea Tree without the Geranium were less active against MRSA. (13)

WHY WOULD ESSENTIAL OILS SUCCEED WHERE ANTIBIOTICS FAIL? THERE IS A CORE DIFFERENCE!

Antibiotics are active due to inhibiting an identifiable single target (a narrow focus). When a microorganism has changed enough to survive the attack of the antibiotic, it will replicate itself freely. Essential oils are fundamentally different. They impair microbes in multiple systems and are non-selective agents (wide and complex vs. a narrow focus) which makes it difficult if not virtually impossible for microorganisms to develop resistance.

The components of essential oils are much wider and varied in focus. In addition, secondary metabolites are made by plants, which contribute to the life and survival of the plant from myriad and various complex environmental attacks. These complex powers are in the essential oils.

SIMPLY PUT: There are many chemical constituents in essential oils vs a simple (one) synthetic antibiotic. Essential oils have hundreds and sometimes even thousands of naturally occurring compounds. Bacteria or microbes simply cannot mutate around all of these complex compounds. And in some cases, microbes are even shut down.

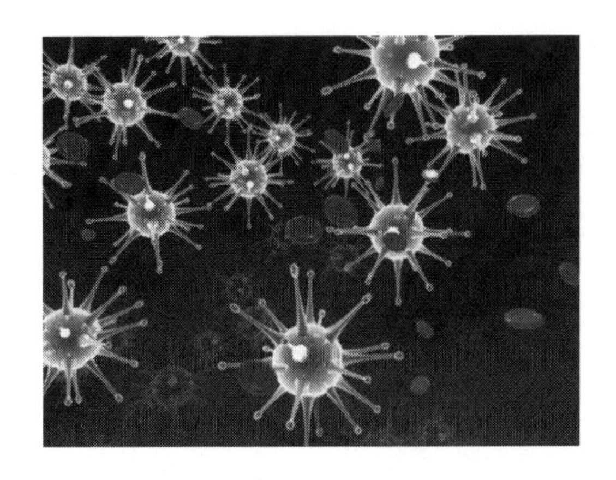

Now, as Robert Tisserand points out, “the single-chemical drug approach has helped to minimize the impact of many diseases, and has saved millions of lives. Pharmaceutical medications are sometimes very effective, and often benefits outweigh risks. But other times the risks seem worse than the benefits, or the medication simply does not work. ADRs (adverse drug reactions) are responsible for an estimated 106,000 deaths in the USA annually (statistics now 10 years old). The increasing widespread use of medication, and of medical intervention, has generated its own set of problems.” (14)

This other set of problems includes not only drug-resistant bacteria and adverse human reactions to drugs but also killing off good bacteria that could lead to poor “gut health”, and conditions like IBS (inflammatory bowel disease) or rheumatoid arthritis, to name a few.

Robert Tisserand sums up the antibiotic issue quite well:
"It seems to be a truism that if you repeatedly try to kill something with a single substance, eventually the 'something' will develop resistance. We see this not only in bacteria, but also in fungi, arthropods (insects, lice, ticks, mites) and cancer cells. It is the principal reason for the corresponding failure of many antibiotic drugs, antifungal drugs, insect repellents and head lice treatments. It is the reason that most chemotherapy protocols now employ more than one drug, and frequently three or four at the same time – single drugs no longer work, because cancer cells have developed resistance to them." (15)

ATTACKING AND ERADICATING BACTERIA AND MICROBES: SOME STUDIES

Let's look first at just a few of the studies on anti-bacterial effects of essential oils. The first was mentioned in the previous chapter.

1) Essential Oils and Future Antibiotics: New Weapons against Emerging "Superbugs"? Nicole Parrish, Nicholas Boire, Stefan Riedel (the authors are with The Johns Hopkins University). Published in the Journal of Ancient Diseases and Preventive Remedies. (16)

Abstract: Antibiotic resistance is emerging at an alarming rate, outpacing current research and development efforts to combat this trend. As a result, many infectious diseases have become difficult to treat; in some cases, no treatment options exist. The search for new antibiotics must accelerate to avoid returning to the 'pre-antibiotic' era.

Ancient remedies, including essential oils and their components, have been explored on a limited basis as a source of new antimicrobials. Many are known to possess significant antimicrobial activity against a wide range of microorganisms. Elucidation of the mechanism of action of these compounds may lead to identification new antibiotic targets. Such targets, once identified, may represent biosynthetic or regulatory pathways not currently inhibited by available drugs. Novel drugs and targets are vital for continued control of infectious diseases worldwide.

"Such investment is not likely to come from the mainstream pharmaceutical industry, which has not placed much emphasis on antibiotic development for a number of reasons, including the excessive cost in bringing a single drug to market without a commensurate return," says Dr. Nicole M. Parrish, associate professor of pathology at the Johns Hopkins University School of Medicine and associate director of medical mycobacteriology at The Johns Hopkins Hospital. (16)

2) Researchers at Cornell University have found lavender essential oil can eradicate certain antibiotic-resistant bacteria, including more than one strain of pathogenic Staphylococcus and pathogenic Streptococcus.

3) In a 1973 study by the German researchers Wagner and Sprinkmeier, a blend of the essential oils of lavender, clove, cinnamon and Melissa (commonly known as lemon balm) was found to be as effective in treating bacterial bronchial conditions as were commercial antibiotics.

Bronchial conditions can also be viral, and studies have determined that lavender oil can effectively disintegrate certain viruses, including flu viruses.

4) Researchers from Australia's Royal Brisbane and Women's Hospital tested a number of plant extracts, including tea tree, lemongrass, and eucalyptus, against several of the most deadly antibiotic-resistant superbugs. These included: Klebsiella pneumonia, MRSA (methicillin-resistant Staphylococcus aureus), VRE (vancomycin-resistant Enterococcus) and more.

They also tested these strains against two common antiseptics often used in hospitals— chlorhexidine and ethanol, commonly termed rubbing alcohol. They then looked at the "zone of inhibition," which is the distance the substance will repel the bug, preventing infection. A larger zone meant the substance was a stronger antiseptic.

RESULTS? Rubbing alcohol had "notably lower or no efficacy in regard to growth inhibition of strains."

- ✓ Lemongrass, eucalyptus, and tea tree oils had large zones of inhibition—significantly greater than the rubbing alcohol.

Lemongrass oil significantly inhibited gram-positive bacteria, while tea tree significantly inhibited gram-negative bacteria. Klebsiella pneumoniae, enterococcus and pseudomonas aeruginosa are all gram-negative bacteria while staphylococcus aureus is a gram-positive bacterium.

The researchers noted, "As proven in vitro, plant-derived antiseptic oils may represent a promising and affordable topical agent to support surgical treatment against multi-resistant and hospital-acquired infections."

5) **The Greek Study**. During the Edinburgh meeting of the Society for General Microbiology, research was presented by representatives from the Technological Educational Institute of Ionian Islands in Greece (17) on the efficacy and health benefits of essential oils and their overall benefits in fighting superbugs (this is the study Dr. Weil commented on earlier in the chapter). The findings were fascinating.

- ✓ Thyme essential oil killed most traces of the drug-resistant bacteria in less than one hour.
- ✓ Cinnamon was nearly as effective against MRSA.

They are well-tolerated and effective against many forms of fungus and bacteria. Essential oils are widely available, says the study, inexpensive, and powerfully effective.

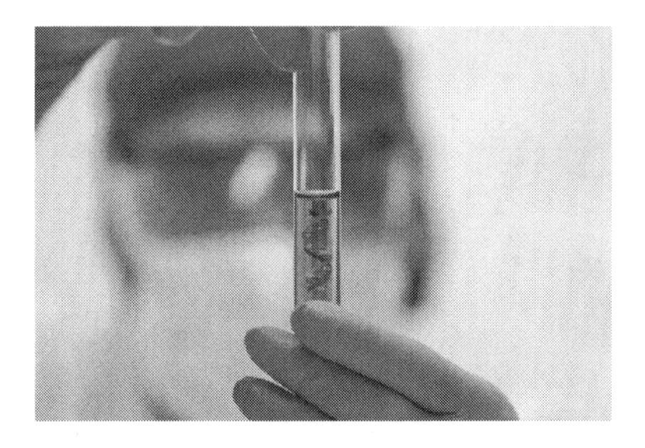

THE DATA FROM THE GREEK INSTITUTE COULDN'T BE ANY MORE CLEAR

Professor Yiannis Samaras explained, "Not only are essential oils a cheap and effective treatment option for antibiotic-resistant strains, but decreased use of antibiotics will help minimize the risk of new strains of antibiotic resistant micro-organisms emerging."

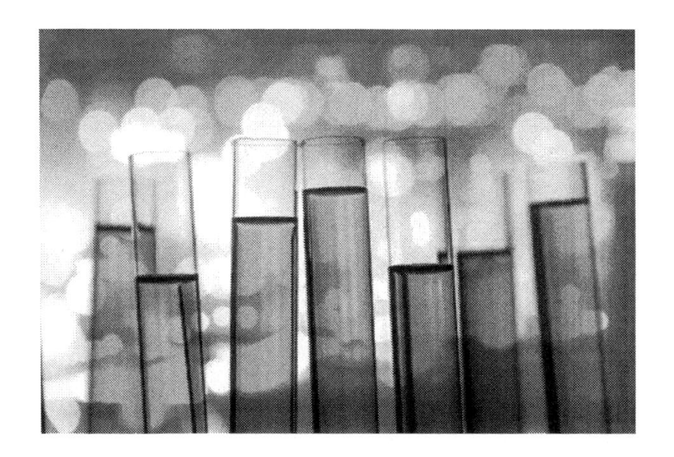

Further information on various anti-bacterial studies noted by the Essential Oils Reference Desk:

- ✓ 1998: Chao studied a blend of oils patterned after that used by 15th century thieves containing cinnamon, rosemary, clove, eucalyptus and lemon was diffused in a closed room in which bacteria cultures were sprayed. There was an 82% reduction in M. Luteus, a 96% reduction in P. Aeruginosa, and a 44% reduction in S Aureus bioaerosols following 10 minutes of exposure.

- ✓ Research published in December 2013 reported that a hand gel made with lemongrass oil was effective in reducing MRSA on the skin of human volunteers, and previous research has shown that a cleanser made with tea-tree oil clears MRSA from the skin as effectively as the standard treatments to which bacteria appear to be developing resistance.

- ✓ Another study compared the effectiveness of essential oils to antibiotics - preliminary results showed cinnamon and oregano are comparable with penicillin and ampicillin in inhibitory activity against e coli and staph aureus.

- ✓ In yet another study with Tea Tree Oil (Melaleuca alternifolia), 30 MRSA (methicillin-resistant Staphylococcus aureus) carriers comparing routine mupirocin nasal ointment and triclosan skin wash with TTO ointment and wash, showed one third were completely cleared by TTO but only 13% by conventional treatment.

- ✓ In a trial with Tea Tree and Herpes cold sores, the oil was found to assist healing to a similar degree as topical 5% acyclovir. Tea Tree oil has about 100 components but 7 terpenes and their related alcohols constitute 80 to 90% of the whole oil. Several of these components have been shown to reduce levels of Staphylococcus aureus and Candida albicans. Terpenes are lipophilic and partition into the phospholipid layer of cell membranes, disrupting normal structure and function. (18)

- ✓ Staph-infected wounds healed faster when they were treated with vapors of tea-tree oil than with conventional methods.

Incorporating essential oils, multi-faceted complex compounds that defy resistance from bacteria, seems the right path. Essential oils can sometimes "turn off", calm or shut down bacteria action and communication, too.

COMBINING ESSENTIAL OILS AND ANTIBIOTICS?

Some studies and research is being done in this area now. The theory is to use the powers of essential oils as explained in this chapter with lower doses of antibiotics, thereby treating the patient, reducing reliance on antibiotics but gleaning its benefits, and reducing costs. I am not a scientist or doctor but feel using antibiotics in this combination doesn't seem right, since antibiotics are part of the problem and include typically synthetic products that can be toxic – but this is pure speculation on my part.

One such study was indeed made in 2012. The paper, "Antibacterial activity of Thymus maroccanus and Thymus broussonetii essential oils against nosocomial infection - bacteria and their synergistic potential with antibiotics" was published by Fadli, Saad A, Sayadi S, Chevalier J, Mezrioui NE, Pagès JM, Hassani L. The summary of results:

> *Out of 80 combinations tested between EOs and antibiotics, 71% showed total synergism, 20% had partial synergistic interaction and 9% showed no effect. Combination with carvacrol, the major constituent of T. maroccanus and T. broussonetii, showed also an interesting synergistic effect in combination with ciprofloxacin. The effect on Gram-positive bacteria was more important than on Gram-negative bacteria. These findings are very*

promising since the use of these combinations for nosocomial infections treatment is likely to reduce the minimum effective dose of the antibiotics, thus minimizing their possible toxic side effects and treatment cost. (19)

Langveld, Veldhuizen and Burt wrote "Synergy between essential oil components and antibiotics: a review." (20) in which they summarize:

With the increase in antibiotic-resistant bacteria and the lack of new antibiotics being brought onto the market, alternative strategies need to be found to cope with infections resulting from drug-resistant bacteria. A possible solution may be to combine existing antibiotics with phytochemicals to enhance the efficacy of antibiotics. A group of phytochemicals that is said to have such effects, according to in vitro studies, is essential oils (EOs) and their components. Amongst others, EOs containing carvacrol, cinnamaldehyde, cinnamic acid, eugenol and thymol can have a synergistic effect in combination with antibiotics. Several modes of action have been put forward by which antibiotics and the essential oil components may act synergistically, such as by affecting multiple targets; by physicochemical interactions and inhibiting antibacterial-resistance mechanisms. Many reported assays show additivity or moderate synergism, indicating that EOs may offer possibilities for reducing antibiotic use.

In the “Open Microbiology Journal”, the scientist-authors of the paper “Essential Oils, A New Horizon in Combating Bacterial Antibiotic Resistance” write a quite detailed and intense analysis review of essential oils. Combining EOs with traditional antibiotics may become a new modality, they write. (21) The review examines the current antibiotic crisis, essential oils that have shown to resist various types of bacteria (see the chart below, printed courtesy the article and its authors), they examine various modalities and issues, discuss the cell wall membrane disturbance and quorum sensing, and conclude:

“Hopefully, the present promising results will open the door for more research into the related field, gain momentum and hasten the process; the discovery will be faster than the evolution of bacteria. The best way is to make full use of the advancement that is available in this era, in the hope that conventional natural products discovery by means of high throughput analysis would shed light on modern drug discovery. Perhaps, in the future, essential oils can progress from being one of the traditional curative agents to become a widely used therapy in the modern medical domain.” (21)

www.ncbi.nlm.nih.gov/pmc/articles/PMC3950955/table/T2/

Table 2.

List of essential oils/antibiotics combinations showing combinatory effects against a panel of microorganisms.

Pair Combinations	Microorganisms	Methods	Interaction	References
Eremanthus erythropappus/ ampicillin	*S. aureus*	Time-kill assay	Synergistic	[37]
Oregano/ fluoroquinolones Oregano/ doxycycline Oregano/ lincomycin Oregano/ maquindox	*E. coli*	Broth microdilution Checkerboard assay	Synergistic	[38]
Pelargonium graveolens/ norfloxacin	*S. aureus, B. cereus*	Agar dilution Checkerboard assay	Synergistic	[30]
Lantana montevidensis/ aminoglycosides	*E. coli*	Broth microdilution Checkerboard assay	Synergistic	[36]
Eugenol/ vancomycin Eugenol/ β-lactams	*E. coli, E. aerogenes, P. vulgaris, P. aeruginosa, S. typhimurium*	Broth microdilution Checkerboard assay	Synergistic	[28]
Croton zehntneri/ gentamicin	*S. aureus, P.aeruginosa*	Disk diffusion test (indirect contact of EO)	-	[37]
Rosmarinus officinalis/ ciprofloxacin	*K. pneumoniae*	Broth microdilution Checkerboard assay	Synergistic	[39]
Eucalyptus/ chlorhexidine digluconate	*Staphylococcus epidermidis*	Broth microdilution Checkerboard assay	Synergistic	[40]
Zataria multiflora/ vancomycin	*S. aureus* (MRSA and MSSA)	Broth microdilution Checkerboard assay	Synergistic	[41]
Aniba rosaeodora/ gentamicin *Pelargonium graveolens*/ gentamicin	*Bacillus cereus, Bacillus subtilis, S. aureus, E. coli, Acinetobacter baumannii, Serratia marcescens, Yersinia enterocolitica*	Broth microdilution Checkerboard assay	Synergistic	[30]
Citrus limon/ amikacin *Cinnamomum zeylanicum*/ amikacin	*Acinetobacter* spp	Broth microdilution Checkerboard assay	Synergistic	[42]

AOL Desktop 9.6 - Connected, Signed-On

Courtesy: Open Microbiol J. 2014; 8: 6–14. Published online 2014 Feb 7. doi: 10.2174/1874285801408010006. Copyright ©

Yap et al.; Licensee Bentham Open. See full charts at the article.

OUR FOOD CHAIN: THE PROBLEM OF LIVESTOCK, ANTIBIOTICS AND SUPERBUGS

Unless we are vegan, we typically consume chicken and red meat. And unless we buy from organic or from highly sensitive-to-the-issues farmers who do not use antibiotics (or only for illness), much of the U.S. livestock is being fed or administered antibiotics. The first antibiotics were given to livestock in 1946 – yes, 1946! – as "growth promoters". (22)

Antibiotics are used to try to keep the animals healthy (especially those in very close quarters) but also to fatten them up more for profits. Part of the issue is that these antibiotics are passed to us and are contributing to poor "gut" health and the antibiotic problem.

Livestock consume up to 80 percent of the antibiotics used in the U.S., writes The Atlantic, and the amount actually jumped by 16 percent between 2009 and 2012 (23) according to a recent FDA report.

This rampant use of the drugs has led in part to the "superbug" problem in that bacterial are becoming increasingly resistant to the antibiotics that are used to treat not just farm animals, but humans as well. In fact, almost 70 percent of the antibiotics given to these animals are classified as "medically important" for humans. (24)

By the way, in 2006 Scandinavia (and the EU) banned antibiotics for use as growth promoters for animals. A report in later 2006 showed a considerable decreased use of antimicrobials in food animal production in Sweden (65%), Denmark (47%), Norway (40%) and Finland (27%). (25) The total use of antibacterial drugs to animals in Sweden decreased by approximately 55% in the period 1986–1999 (they had started to decrease before the ban.) Further, the ban of growth promoters in Europe and Scandinavia demanded the improvement of the hygiene of farms.

It was shown that under good production conditions it is possible to reach good and competitive production results for the rearing of poultry without the continuous use of antibiotics in feeds. (26)

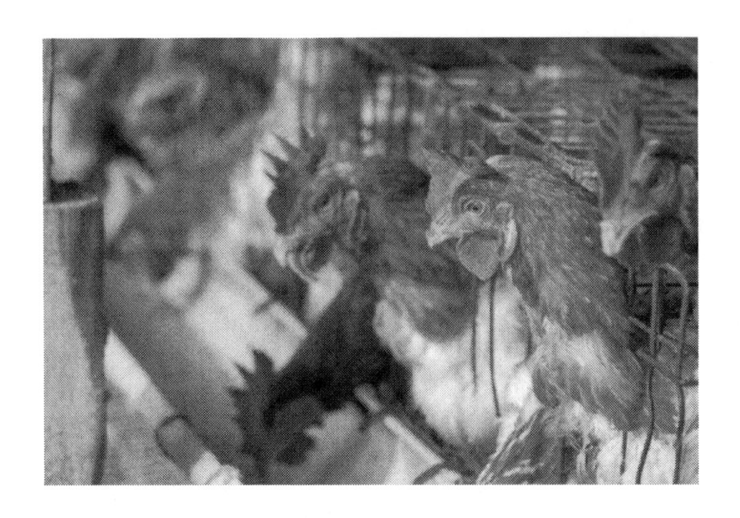

Now back to the U.S.

Writes Dr. Mercola (27), “Attempts by the Food and Drug Administration (FDA) to decrease the widespread use of antibiotics in livestock production have seldom succeeded...In 2014, the FDA again tried to regulate antibiotics [after previous attempts], floating a new plan in which drug makers voluntarily agree to remove “growth promotion and feed efficiency” as approved uses on livestock antibiotic labels so the drugs would only be used in cases of sickness and under the care of veterinarians.

While drug makers have until the end of 2016 to make the voluntary changes, so far results are very disappointing and use of antibiotics has actually gone up rather than down.

Mercola continues in the same article:

> *While antibiotic resistance can result from natural adaptation, it "is exacerbated by inappropriate use of pharmaceuticals, and the prevalence of resistance in the agricultural sector is generally higher in animal species reared under intensive production systems," says the United Nations Food and Agriculture Organization (FAO).*
>
> *The risk of resistance "appears to be particularly high in countries where legislation, surveillance, prevention and monitoring are weak or inadequate," says FAO Deputy Director-General Helena Semedo. The routine and indiscriminate use of antibiotics in livestock production has produced "superbugs" that can create life-threatening diseases for humans because the drugs we have relied upon for years no longer work.*

"Most people have heard of MRSA and the dread gut bacterium Clostridium difficile, but clinicians increasingly worry about vancomycin-resistant enterococci (VRE), and resistant Acinetobacter baumannii — which so plagued US troops in Iraq it was called 'Iraqibacter.'

Klebsiella pneumoniae carbapenemase (KPC) and a family of bugs called Carbapenem-resistant Enterobacteriaceae (CRE) are also growing. KPC broke out in the nation's top research hospitals, the Clinical Center at the National Institutes of Health in Bethesda, in 2011 killing 12. MRSA caused a well-publicized infection in Giants tight end Daniel Fells and has been reported found on public beaches by Florida researchers."

Recently, scientists have discovered a gene in bacteria that helps them develop this quick resistance to even last-resort antibiotics. Called the MCR-1 gene, it has been found in pigs and humans in China and other countries including Canada though not yet in the US says the Scientific American. The gene likely originated in livestock, but has now been found in human bacterial samples as well.

[In addition] by killing 'good' bacteria with important roles in the body, 'Overuse of antibiotics could be fueling the dramatic increase in conditions such as obesity, Type 1 diabetes, inflammatory bowel disease, allergies and asthma. (27)

DR. STUART LEVY ON ANTIBIOTICS AND LIVESTOCK

As reported in The Atlantic (28), Dr. Stuart B. Levy is a man of many titles—hematologist and professor at Tufts University; director of the Center for Adaptation, Genetics, and Drug Resistance; president of the Alliance for the Prudent Use of Antibiotics; and author of the book "The Antibiotic Paradox: How the Misuse of Antibiotics Destroys Their Curative Powers". He and his colleagues consider the misuse of antibiotics on farms to be the biggest influence on antibiotic resistance, which has been declared "an increasingly serious threat to global public health that requires action across all government sectors and society".

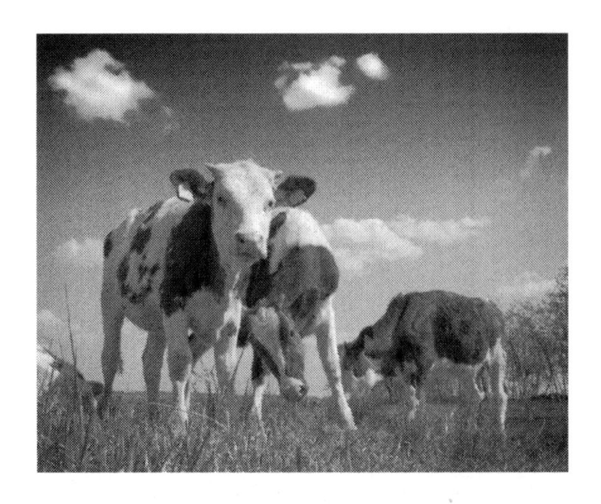

Levy has been warning about this impending disaster for nearly 40 years, a couple of decades after farmers discovered that putting small amounts of antibiotics in the animals' feed resulted in increased growth.

Even back then, a study led by Levy found that chickens developed resistance to the antibiotic tetracycline at a rapid pace–within a week, the animals had resistant bacteria in their gut. Months later, the stubborn bugs had spread to untreated chickens and even the farmers.

And it didn't stop there: Those resistant bacteria also became resistant to other antibiotics that the chickens hadn't even consumed. "Antibiotics used anywhere creates antibiotic resistance, and that resistance doesn't stay in that environment," Levy says. "And resistance is transferrable among bacteria of different types."

WHAT TO DO?

In 2014, as previously mentioned, the FDA tried again (after a number of efforts) to regulate antibiotics, whereby drug makers voluntarily agree to remove "growth promotion and feed efficiency" as approved uses on livestock antibiotic labels – meaning the antibiotics could only be used under the care of vets for real illness. This seems difficult to regulate.

There has been resistance, lobbyists and agricultural groups trying to block the FDA actions, and frankly oversight will be tough. What is really needed is that farmers should understand WHY and HOW this is a crisis, and to "buy in" to be part of the solution. Money and economics is surely a factor, but the future of our health is a bigger factor. And there is a strong alternative on the horizon.

ESSENTIAL OILS FOR LIVESTOCK

The following is from the excellent research and several articles written by Cari Romm and Tori Rodriguez of The Atlantic (29, 30):

Numerous recent studies—including several done by the USDA—have shown great promise in using essential oils as an alternative to antibiotics in livestock. One of their studies, published in October 2014 in the journal Poultry Science, found that chickens that consumed feed with added oregano oil had a 59 percent lower mortality rate due to ascites, a common infection in poultry, than untreated chickens.

Other research, from a 2011 issue of BMC Proceedings, showed that adding a combination of plant extracts—from oregano, cinnamon, and chili peppers—actually changed the gene expression of treated chickens, resulting in weight gain as well as protection against an injected intestinal infection. A 2010 study from Poultry Science produced similar findings with the use of extracts from turmeric, chili pepper, and shiitake mushrooms. A multi-year study is currently underway at the USDA that includes investigations into the use of citrus peels and essential oils as drug alternatives.

Researchers have also directly compared the effects of commonly used antibiotics with those of various essential oils. One such study, from the March 2012 issue of the Journal of Animal Science, found that rosemary and oregano oils resulted in the same amount of growth in chickens as the antibiotic avilamycin, and that the oils killed bacteria, too. Additional findings have shown that essential oils help reduce salmonella in chickens, and another study found that a blend of several oils can limit the spread of salmonella among animals.

One of the co-authors of that study, Dr. Charles Hofacre, a professor at the University of Georgia's College of Veterinary Medicine, says it's such a new area of research that they don't yet know exactly how the essential oils work, but "there is some strong evidence that they are functioning by both an antibacterial action in the intestine and also some have an effect to stimulate the intestinal cells ability to recover from disease more quickly–either by local immunity or helping keep the intestinal cells themselves healthier." (31)

POULTRY AND CARGILL

Cargill researchers are focusing on improving gut health in poultry to promote feed efficiency and keep birds healthy. (32) A major corporation, Cargill has been researching the use of non-medicated feed additives for several years as an alternative to antibiotic growth promoters (AGPs). They write:

> As an independent supplier, Cargill has performed cross-additive research and determined the most beneficial types of feed additives for individual customer needs. For consistent performance improvement, essential oils turned out to be a key solution because they impact all four key gut function areas.
>
> Since 2009, a combined total of 77 comprehensive in vitro and in vivo trials have been conducted at Cargill's Animal Nutrition Innovation Centers in Velddriel, the Netherlands, and Elk River, Minn., as well as at regional facilities in Jordan, France, Poland, India and the U.S., on additives including essential oils, probiotics, yeast derivatives and medium chain fatty acids (MCFA).
>
> ESSENTIAL OILS AND GUT HEALTH
>
> Cargill seeks to better understand optimal gut function in four key areas:

1) Managing microflora for a well-balanced bacterial population
2) Controlling immune function and inflammatory response
3) Maximizing nutrient digestion and absorption
4) Improving the physical barrier against pathogens

While all additives studied showed some benefit in these areas, Cargill researchers found that selected essential oil compounds, particularly those derived from thyme, cinnamon and oregano, had the most comprehensive effect on overall gut health.

Benefits included:

- ✓ Antimicrobial activity
- ✓ Modulation of immune response
- ✓ Antioxidant activity
- ✓ Improvement of nutrient digestibility
- ✓ Stimulation of mucus production

"Only essential oils have both a broad spectrum of activity against pathogens and a direct impact on digestive function," said Stephanie Ladirat, global technology lead for gut health additives in Cargill's animal nutrition business.

Long-term Benefits of Healthy Digestion in Poultry

For poultry producers the high return on investment is a top benefit of intestinal health support. However, promoting gut health also helps address issues in food safety and animal welfare. Healthy poultry intestines may result in a lower risk of bacterial food contamination and in healthier barn environments.

Finally, feed efficiency has become increasingly important due to the growing world population and limitations in feed resources. Supporting gut heath contributes to efforts to meet increasing demand for global animal protein in an efficient way. "Promoting gut health while reducing AGPs is critical for sustainable animal performance and profitability," adds Van Gerwe. "Our R&D work in improving poultry gut health is an important part of Cargill's commitment to nourishing the world's population."

In March of 2016, Cargill announced that it is eliminating 20 percent of shared-class antibiotics, those deemed important for human medicine and farm animals, from its four feed yards in Texas, Kansas and Colorado, and four additional feed yards operated by Friona Industries, which is a strategic business partner that supplies the company with cattle.

The issue of our antibiotic crisis, the fact that big pharma can no longer just "make a new antibiotic that works", and our serious consequences for future wellness are at stake.

Essential oils should play a role in the solution for both humans and livestock.

As Aminov wrote, in summary: "The current state in the field of antimicrobials, resistance, and chemotherapy is certainly not limited to clinical microbiology as it was in the early years of the antibiotic era. Thus, it is not a single grand challenge; it is rather a complex problem requiring concerted efforts of microbiologists, ecologists, health care specialists, educationalists, policy makers, legislative bodies, agricultural and pharmaceutical industry workers, and the public to deal with. In fact, this should be of everyone's concern, because, in the end, there is always a probability for any of us at some stage to get infected with a pathogen that is resistant to antibiotic treatment." (33)

Let's take a look at why there has been somewhat of a barrier to medical or therapeutic applications of essential oils in the U.S. in the next chapter.

Chapter 5

DIFFERENT APPROACHES TO ESSENTIAL OILS AROUND THE WORLD

Be curious, not judgmental. ~ Walt Whitman

Aromatherapy and the use of essential oils vary from country to country and culture to culture. You already have a taste of this from previous chapters, including history and research. Let's take a deeper look.

In Great Britain, much of Europe, Australia, Canada and the Far East, trained aromatherapists study physiology, science, massage techniques, properties of essential oils and how to use them, as well as blend them, for client's needs. Essential oils and the modality of massage is a far more accepted practice for everyday health – but there are even differences between these countries.

It is not disputed in the U.S. that fragrance can affect emotion and mood, however its value for healing "does not resonate well with Western pharmacology. It appears that drug-development-oriented pharmacology would just as well not even deal with the phenomenon of fragrance..." (1)

Dr Kurt Schnaubelt wrote, in "The Healing Intelligence of Essential Oils":

> It is a defining problem of conventional medicine that realities that defy reductionist interpretation are treated as nonexistent. In silent conspiracy, the industry acts as if such phenomena simply do not exist. "It is impossible that Lavender heals burns, because there is no research." (2)
>
> "...Pharmacology is forced to pick a (presumed) active ingredient and to measure its effect, if for no other reason than to keep the number of experiments manageable. One has to conclude that the active ingredient concept does not arise from observing specific activity but is instead

> maintained so the reductionist process makes sense.
>
> Using Lavender as a remedy for burns is again the classic example. It is highly effective, but only within the Aromatherapy community. U.S. pharmacology does not recommend the use of Lavender, since it cannot find an active ingredient that mimics the effect of the whole oil." (2)

The antibacterial activity of essential oils has been acknowledged through the ages, written about throughout history (remember those clay tablets, Greek & Roman scholars, the Leech Book of Bald, etc.) and studied scientifically since the 1900s.

There have been numerous studies (especially in France) that show how strong they are against bacteria and microbes. Dr. Valnet and others, including Paul Belaiche, have written on this (Belaiche in the 1970s). Yet in the U.S. the line is that they can't be taken seriously because not much study has been done, and essential oils have been disregarded. (I have tried to demonstrate in Chapter 3 that there is indeed a growing body of research on the subject with just a sampling of research.)

Dr. Schnaubelt wrote in "Medical Aromatherapy" that "the concepts of reductionist experimentation have taken on such a dominance that only those realities open to this mode of experimentation are considered real. Phenomena too complex for this method are arrogantly declared irrelevant."

Reductionist theory: Biologists often use scientific reductionism, focusing on 1 component at a time. However, many opponents attack the process, believing that biological organisms are too complex to explain by numbers or single parts alone. It stands as a vast oversimplification.

Even physicists are finding that the quest for fundamental particles making up matter and governing the laws of the universe may be much too difficult to study, without looking at the model as a whole.

So bringing this argument to essential oils and medical applications as well as a more established view in the U.S. that has held essential oils back:

Unlike antibiotics, which are active due to inhibiting an easily identifiable single target and single action, the activity of essential oils – impairing bacteria in multiple physiological systems as well as in membrane functionality, is complex, wide and numerous. By trying to apply a reductionist theory to essential oils defeats the purpose.

LET'S LOOK AT DIFFERENT SCHOOLS OF AROMATHERAPY AND HOW DIFFERENT COUNTRIES HAVE EVOLVED

The Atlantic Institute of Aromatherapy shared very interesting information about the different "schools" of aromatherapy (though some in the industry don't agree with this):

The separation of aromatherapy methods into "schools" really began in the early 2000s when one of Dr. Daniel Pénoël's lectures included a joke that manifested.

Dr. Pénoël, whose speaking style is very charismatic and humorous, described the differences between the three schools in this way:

"The German system of aromatherapy is comparable to platonic love. You cannot make babies with platonic love. The English system is like flirting. You still cannot make babies. The French system of aromatherapy is like 'The Full Monty,' and it will make babies!" (4)

The contention is that the differences in aromatherapy paths between France, Germany and the U.S. are rooted in history. All styles believe in natural essential oil powers for treatment and betterment of health, but the way it has been accepted and viewed "mainstream" are indeed different.

French-Style Medical Aromatherapy

First and foremost, fragrance and plant-based usage has a deep history in France, especially in the south of France, as we have witnessed throughout this book and especially in the history section. (The south of France and specifically Grasse are also in the global forefront for the perfume industry.) The south of France already had a name for itself and lavender early on. Plants were processed in the 11th century to improve the odor of leather made locally in tanneries. The international strength of the perfume industry in the south surely had a part in the development of aromatherapy and use of essential oils.

Even before Gattefosse turned his attention and life devotion to aromatherapy and published his first book in 1937, others were researching the work and there are clear pre-cursors who helped his path. Chemists Charabot and Dupont were classifying the components of essential oils and researching therapeutic uses (which Gattefosse elaborated on.)

"Original French-style aromatherapy focused on the treatment of infections," writes Schnaubelt. In the French perspective, aromatherapy is a medical method to treat disease with essential oils, and it was used, applied and practiced by physicians (unlike in the U.S. for instance.) (5) The Atlantic Institute continues:

> As medicinal aromatherapy took root, it began to engage pharmacists, chemists and physicians in France and all over Europe; however, many were in France. In 1978, Dr. Paul Belaiche published on the clinical use of essential oils in treatment of infectious and degenerative diseases. Belaiche was an MD, and he

combined clinical application with in-vitro research on the beneficial effects of essential oils. One important study he conducted and wrote about showed oregano, clove, thyme, tea tree and cinnamon to have the special wide antibacterial and antifungal properties.

Jean-Claude Lapraz, Christian Duraffourd, and Dominique Baudoux have all contributed enormously to the understanding of the medical activity of essential oils, as well. In 1980, French chemist Henri Viaud published the purity and quality criteria that essential oils have to meet to be suitable for medical purposes. Then, in the 1990s, Dr. Daniel Pénoël and Pierre Franchomme contributed the medical aroma text of the decade.

The contributions of these French and Belgian doctors and pharmacists have greatly added to the understanding of how to incorporate essential oils into medical treatments. This has become known as the "French method."

In France, it is illegal for anyone other than a physician or registered pharmacist to administer essential oils therapeutically. The French-style often uses essential oils undiluted, or neat. In addition, French-style sometimes includes ingesting essential oils or use in suppositories. Therapies are developed understanding the body, chemistry and pharmacology, often with lab tests.

The medical community embraced and accepted the powers of essential oils, and this has made a difference in how the uses have progressed.

United Kingdom

British-style aromatherapy started to take off in the 1950s with Marguerite Maury, as we read, and it came to the forefront in the 1980s. There was a strong and renewed interest, and it caught on with the public. Much of this early modern audience followed Robert Tisserand's book "The Art of Aromatherapy", by the way, and then tons of information proliferated at all levels.

The British-style tends to use dilutions with lots of carrier oils, and favors massage therapy. In the U.K., the non-academic and non-medical communities were the early enthusiasts, and a certain amount of antagonism and doubt surfaced from the medical circles, who spoke of the lack of "science" and did not initially embrace essential oils as they did in France. However, that has changed.

It is today considered a "complementary therapy" that can help to promote relaxation. It is currently widely used in the management of chronic pain, depression, anxiety and stress, insomnia and some cognitive disorders.

In the U.K., complementary and alternative medicine (CAM) includes a group of diverse medical and healthcare systems, practices and products that are not generally considered part of conventional medicine. Complementary medicine is generally regarded as additional treatment that is used alongside conventional medicine, whereas alternative medicine is regarded as a treatment used in place of conventional medicine. Aromatherapy is regarded as complementary medicine. (6)

A report in The Lancet in 2007 stated that about 13,000 patients had been treated at four homeopathic hospitals (Bristol, Glasgow, Liverpool and London) in the UK each year. 14.5% of the population say that they trust homeopathy and £38 million is spent on homeopathy each year in the UK. (7)

Aromatherapy certainly flourishes today in the form of massage therapy as a modality, as used by the general population.

Switzerland

Dana Ullman did extensive reporting on a big health move in Switzerland, whereby homeopathic treatments and complimentary alternative methods (CAM) can be reimbursed by the national health insurance program following a comprehensive publication of homeopathic medicine. This is on a test basis to 2018, when it will be evaluated again. Dana writes: (8)

> *In late 2011, the Swiss government's report on homeopathic medicine represents the most comprehensive evaluation of homeopathic medicine ever written by a government and was just published in book form in English (Bornhoft and Matthiessen, 2011). This breakthrough report affirmed that homeopathic treatment is both effective and cost-effective and that*

homeopathic treatment should be reimbursed by Switzerland's national health insurance program.

The Swiss government's inquiry into homeopathy and complementary and alternative (CAM) treatments resulted from the high demand and widespread use of alternatives to conventional medicine in Switzerland, not only from consumers but from physicians as well. Approximately half of the Swiss population have used CAM treatments and value them. Further, about half of Swiss physicians consider CAM treatments to be effective. Perhaps most significantly, 85 percent of the Swiss population wants CAM therapies to be a part of their country's health insurance program.

It is therefore not surprising that more than 50 percent of the Swiss population surveyed prefer a hospital that provides CAM treatments rather to one that is limited to conventional medical care.

Beginning in 1998, the government of Switzerland decided to broaden its national health insurance to include certain complementary and alternative medicines, including homeopathic medicine, traditional Chinese medicine, herbal medicine, anthroposophic medicine, and neural therapy. This reimbursement was provisional while the Swiss government commissioned an extensive study on these treatments to determine if they were effective and cost-effective. The provisional reimbursement for these alternative treatments ended in 2005, but as a result of this new study, the Swiss government's health insurance program once again began to reimburse for homeopathy and select alternative treatments. In fact, as a result of a national referendum in which more than two-thirds of voters supported the inclusion of homeopathic and select alternative medicines in Switzerland's national health care insurance program, the field of complementary and alternative medicine has become a part of this government's constitution (Dacey, 2009; Rist, Schwabl, 2009).

The Swiss government's "Health Technology Assessment" on homeopathic medicine is much more comprehensive than any previous governmental report written on this subject to date. Not only did this report carefully and comprehensively review the body of evidence from randomized double-blind and placebo controlled clinical trials testing homeopathic medicines, they also evaluated the "real world effectiveness" as well as safety and cost-effectiveness.

The report also conducted a highly-comprehensive review of the wide body of preclinical research (fundamental physio-chemical research, botanical studies, animal studies, and in vitro studies with human cells).

And still further, this report evaluated systematic reviews and meta-analyses, outcome studies, and epidemiological research. This wide review carefully evaluated the studies conducted, both in terms of quality of design and execution (called "internal validity") and how appropriate each was for the way that homeopathy is commonly practiced (called "external validity"). The subject of external validity is of special importance because some scientists and physicians conduct research on homeopathy with little or no understanding of this type of medicine (some studies tested a homeopathic medicine that is rarely used for the condition tested, while others utilized medicines not commonly indicated for specific patients). When such studies inevitably showed that the homeopathic medicine did not "work," the real and accurate assessment must be that the studies were set up to disprove homeopathy... or simply, the study was an exploratory trial that sought to evaluate the results of a new treatment (exploratory trials of this nature are not meant to prove or disprove the system of homeopathy but only to evaluate that specific treatment for a person with a specific condition).

After assessing pre-clinical basic research and the high quality clinical studies, the Swiss report affirmed that homeopathic high-potencies seem to induce regulatory effects (e.g., balancing or normalizing effects) and specific changes in cells or living organisms. The report also reported that 20 of the 22 systematic reviews of clinical research testing homeopathic medicines *detected at least a trend in favor of homeopathy.* (Bornhöft, Wolf, von Ammon, et al, 2006)*

The Swiss report found a particularly strong body of evidence to support the homeopathic treatment of Upper Respiratory Tract Infections and Respiratory Allergies. The report cited 29 studies in "Upper Respiratory Tract Infections/AllergicReactions," of which 24 studies found a positive result in favor of homeopathy. Further, six out of seven controlled studies that compared homeopathic treatment with conventional medical treatment showed that homeopathy to be more effective than conventional medical interventions (the one other trial found homeopathic treatment to be equivalent to conventional medical treatment). All of these results from homeopathic treatment came without the side effects common to conventional drug treatment. In evaluating only the randomized placebo controlled trials, 12 out of 16 studies showed a positive result in favor of homeopathy.

The bottom line is that large numbers of the Swiss population use homeopathic medicines and select other natural therapies. After a nationwide referendum in May 2009 that found a two-thirds majority (!) favoring the integration of CAM into the Swiss health system, the Swiss Minister of Health approved reimbursement by the government's health program for five leading natural therapies, including anthroposophic medicine, homeopathy, neural therapy, phytotherapy/herbal medicine, and traditional Chinese medicine, for a test period until 2018.

German Style

Use of essential oils in Germany focuses on inhalation and diffusing. Certainly homeopathic approaches and alternative treatments like essential oils are used and acknowledged. It is estimated that more than 1.5 million patients per year are treated in Germany homeopathically or with alternative care (such as with aromatherapy).

Essential oils are dispensed by physicians for therapeutic use in Germany.

As we learned in the history section of this book, aromatherapy is rooted in history. A German physician, Hieronymus Braunschweig, wrote several books on essential oil distillation which went through hundreds of editions in every European language. As early as 1597, he referenced 25 essential oils including rosemary, lavender, clove, cinnamon, myrrh, and nutmeg for wellness uses.

United States

The route in the U.S. is similar to the U.K. Many people discovered (or are discovering) essential oils and aromatherapy, but the pharmacy and medical communities were (or are) hostile or non-accepting in general (though this is changing.)

Paraphrasing from Dr. Schnaubelt's various writings on the subject: *On one side is big pharma and the HMO "industry" grossing trillions of dollars in the U.S. Corporations convince citizens that drugs and medical procedures are the most effective, reasonable and best way to cure disease, while on the other side are humans who might wish to try alternative routes of healing. More and more Americans are visiting alternative therapists and more doctors are moving to an integrated approach.*

Some of this is rooted in the history of the U.S., when holistic and natural medicine was growing in popularity but the established medical world was hostile and fighting against it. An interesting piece by Dana Ullman shows the hostility even to President Abraham Lincoln who followed holistic medicine.

> *The public today does not adequately understand the degree of animosity that conventional doctors had toward homeopathic physicians. The reasoning for this animosity is probably best described in the words of one doctor to an AMA meeting:*
>
> *"Too many wives of conventional physicians are going to homeopathic physicians. And to make it worse," he added, "they are taking their children to homeopaths too."*
>
> *Homeopathic physicians were not simply competitors to conventional physicians;*

homeopaths were medically trained and could not be considered "uneducated" or under-educated. Further, inherent in homeopathy is a profound respect for the "wisdom of the body," and therefore, homeopaths tend to maintain a significant skepticism of and criticism for using powerful drug treatments that tend to suppress symptoms and push a person's disease deeper into his/her body and mind.

The conventional medical community was also threatened by the fact that homeopathy was attracting so many U.S. cultural leaders. The strongest advocates for homeopathy tended to be educated classes and wealthy Americans as well as the abolitionists, the literary greats (including virtually all of the leading American transcendentalist authors), and the suffragists (homeopaths admitted women into their medical schools and associations several decades before the conventional doctors did).

In the 19th century, the AMA did not enforce the many ethical code or professional health care violations of its members, therefore allowing physicians to prescribe mercury in dangerously high doses, enabling physicians to blood-let their patients to death, and even engage in treatment while inebriated. And yet, the AMA was ridiculously strict in their enforcement of their ethical code against any interaction with homeopathic doctors or their patients.

One AMA member got kicked out of his local medical society for consulting with a homeopath who also happened to be his wife.

Typhoid fever caused more deaths during the Civil War and the Spanish-American War than the deaths caused by bullets. History shows that homeopathy gained widespread popularity in the United States and Europe from its successes in treating various infectious disease epidemics of the mid- and late-1800s, including typhoid epidemics. Despite these good results, the AMA's influence on governmental regulations led to stipulation that graduates of homeopathic medical colleges could not receive a military commission.

Thankfully, the antagonism toward homeopaths was not as severe during World War I; almost 2,000 homeopathic physicians were commissioned as medical officers. Even the American Red Cross authorized a homeopathic hospital unit.

Recent research has confirmed the clinical efficacy of homeopathic medicines and the cost-effectiveness of homeopathic treatment, as determined by what is widely recognized as the most comprehensive report ever conducted on homeopathy -- and this report was commissioned by the government of Switzerland. (9)

I included this information to show the differences of what was occurring in a place like France, with medical doctors and scientists fully behind essential oils, conducting research, recognizing the inherent powers and writing on it, with a general acceptance of not only the medical and scientific world but the public. Contrast that to what was occurring in the U.S. and you can see how the differences are rooted.

The embedded views of the "traditional" medical world, pharmaceutical lobby as well as corporate insurance and the legal world have held back a more common usage of essential oils (and other natural therapies) in the U.S., though this is changing. Some U.S. hospitals are now employing aromatherapy, more doctors are considering it or integrating it into their practices, we are seeing more integrative practices, and more of the general public is becoming aware of the natural power of essential oils.

I am not hostile to the medical world and great advances and people who have taken their part in history; I am disappointed and hostile to those in the medical world who do not understand or believe that alternative, natural therapies have their place in our world. I am hostile to just fixing a symptom (which might not need fixing) with a pill that may or may not include elements "poisonous" to the system, instead of finding the source of the problem, as the alternative and Ayurvedic worlds do; and not understanding the key links between mind, body and soul in our overall health.

Following the key phrase “Do no harm” – certain drugs and invasive procedures do not follow this credo.

Chinese Approach

China has a long history of plant-based, herbal medicine. There is quite a difference between the Eastern and Western approach toward treating disease. In fact, the Chinese view is to treat the individual not the disease per se – and this is more similar to the Ayurvedic approach as well. Western medicine tends to treat the symptoms of a disease (not the underlying cause) and applies the same medicine to the same disease. The Chinese approach is that symptoms are not primarily caused by the original microbe but are manifested by how the body is responding to it. The same disease could be treated in different ways in different people – you treat the person, not the disease.

Chinese medicine believes that essential oils interact with the yuan | original qi to influence the disease processes. They often connect essential oils and their qualities to the five elements to deal with excess or deficiency (i.e. excess water, fire deficiency).

According to Taoist master Jeffrey Yuen (and written about by Dr. Schnaubelt), Chinese traditional medicine looks at the main characteristic of an essential oil to determine its therapeutic application.

Juxtapositioning the outlooks, the Western medical world tends to focus on the molecular structures of drugs, and how a specific drug performs in research to treat a condition. The Chinese view is not concerned with the molecular structure but with its function or character. Meaning, it recognizes the healing properties of plants without making any statement about the active ingredient or molecular structure. This is closer to the Ayurvedic approach as well.

CHAPTER 6

MIND – BODY – SPIRIT AND AROMATHERAPY

"One fact remains: from time immemorial, in every country, aromatic plants have always been considered the most effective treatment for diseases afflicting mankind... This is not because, as some believe, the smell attracts the attention of the uninitiated better and stimulate auto-suggestion in the patient, but rather because volatile aromatic substances have true therapeutic value."
~ Rene-Maurice Gattefossé

Aromatherapy is the use of essential oils for psychological and physical well-being. Gattefossé coined the term, but aromatherapy dates back thousands of years. Aromatherapy treats the emotional, physical and spiritual health, that is, mind-body-spirit. The intentions of the oils are to heal the body and mind.

Aromatherapy can be used for medical applications

(such as healing a burn or wound, for anti-bacterial applications, bringing down inflammation, attacking bacteria, help a chemotherapy patient with nausea, etc.)

Aromatherapy can be used for wellness applications (helping one to sleep restfully, calming an anxiety attack, helping one focus, helping with grief, improving the immune system, in a therapeutic massage, etc.)

Aromatherapy can be used for "environmental atmosphere" (such as diffusing scents to create an inviting, grounded or energetic room; calm patients in a dentist-office, as well as purifying the air of microbes.)

The bottom line is that essential oils can penetrate not only the blood-brain barrier, but they can also penetrate the skin, follow nerve pathways, follow the meridians, and provide healing and balance even at the cellular level such as cellular memory and limbic system (that emotional control center.)

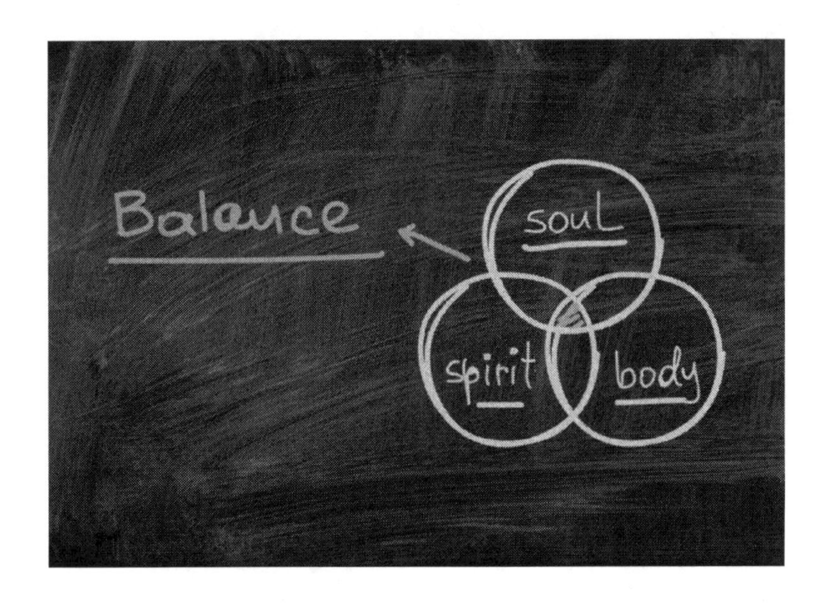

MIND AND BODY ARE INTERCONNECTED

Our mind and body are powerful allies. How you think can affect how you feel. And how you feel can affect your thinking. Energy is related to this – we are in fact energy beings.

An example of this mind-body connection is how your body responds to stress. Constant worry and stress over jobs, finances, children, spousal illness, death in the family or other problems can cause tense muscles, pain, headaches, and stomach problems. It may also lead to high blood pressure or other serious problems. Your mind and the situation around you cause the stress – your body responds.

On the other hand, constant pain or a health problem like heart disease or arthritis can affect your emotions. You might become depressed, anxious, and stressed, which could affect how well you treat, manage, or cope with your illness. In this case your body is causing the problem which is then translated to your emotions and mind.

Pessimism promotes ill health, and it can shorten your life.

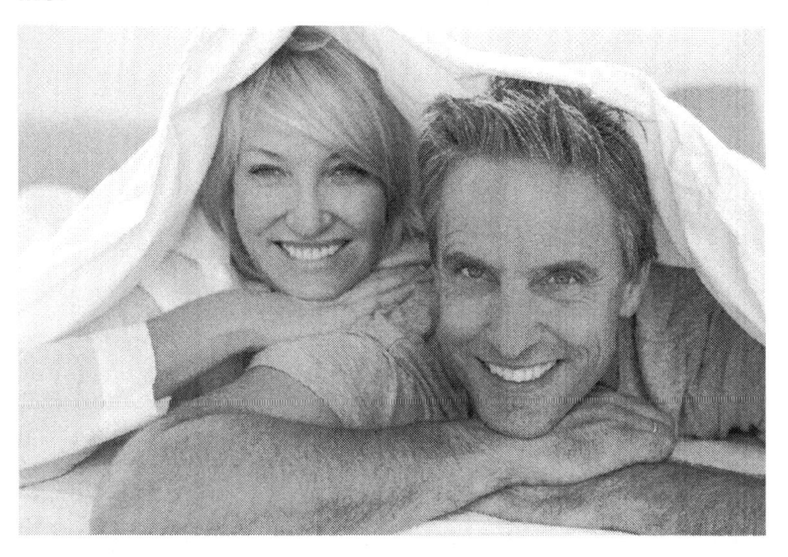

But your mind can have a positive effect on your

health, too. Having a positive outlook on life might help you better handle pain, stress or illness, and stay healthier than someone who is less hopeful. Optimists have more T-helper cells in their immune systems than pessimists. Optimists suffer only half the number of infections pessimists do.

There are innumerable stories of couples who have been married for a long time – one dies, and the other may pass soon afterward, even if he or she was not ill. The mind and soul were affected deeply, hearts were broken to the extreme. This is a phenomenon known as "broken heart" syndrome, says Dr. Mark Hyman. He says the New England Journal of Medicine published a study about how grief or emotional trauma can cause heart failure — literally, a broken heart and psyche. (1)

Research shows that during the first week after the death of a spouse, mortality skyrockets to double the normal rate. (2)

Poor emotional health can affect the immune system and your overall wellness.

GENES AFFECTED BY EMOTIONS? I THOUGHT THEY WERE FIXED & FINITE?

And this is mind-blowing but not well-known: "Cellular biologist Bruce Lipton, PhD., is one of the leading authorities on how emotions can regulate genetic expression, which are explained in-depth in his excellent books "The Biology of Belief, and Spontaneous Evolution." (3)

What he is saying is that your genes are affected by your response or reaction to your conscious thoughts, emotions, and unconscious beliefs. (This is related to the newer field of epigenetics, how your genes can affect your DNA and that of your children, which I write about later in the chapter.)

So in other words, while traditional science told us that we are a "victim" of our genetics and family history, newer science is telling us we can take control and affect our health or illness by not only our environment and choices (like diet) but also by our thoughts and emotions.

This is why a holistic approach to the mind (emotional health) and the body (diet, exercise, physical care) is so important for wellness and balance, and why aromatherapy can be powerfully helpful. Essential oils help balance emotional health (which helps with the body) and can help with physical care (which helps with the mind or emotion.)

Today, the World Health Organization (WHO) estimates that 65-80% of the population is now using holistic naturopathic medicine as a primary form of health care. Many are on to something.

By the say, in ancient Greece, three doctors would see the patient together. They were the "knife" doctor, the "herb" doctor, and the "word" doctor. The modern day counterparts (surgeon, internist and psychiatrist) rarely see a patient together, let alone even speak together. (4)

HOW DOES AROMATHERAPY PLAY INTO THIS?

Inhaled essential oils go DIRECTLY to the limbic

system, are interpreted and the brain sends instructions. Using the example of stress and cortisol again, certain essential oils (rosemary among them) BRING DOWN cortisol levels thereby helping someone who is stressed or experiencing an anxiety attack to relax.

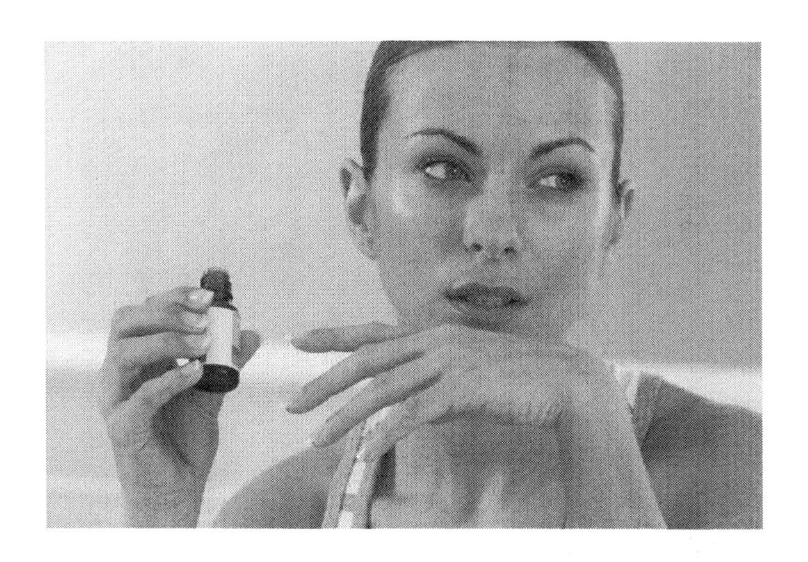

Certain essential oil constituents encourage focus or memory – when the aroma comes to the limbic system, the hippocampus or other areas of the brain are aided or instructed what to do. Someone having trouble falling asleep could inhale lavender essential oil to help bring on a restful sleep. Lavender increases slow-wave sleep, the very deep stage in which the heartbeat slows and muscles relax – among other powers. During this phase, the brain is thought to organize memory. It is the mind AND body that are affected and aided in all of these cases.

Certain essential oils can support the adrenal glands or stimulate the immune system; others (like lemon) excel at eliminating toxins and supporting white blood cells that fight infection; almost all have anti-bacterial qualities that can help support the immune system by knocking out pathogens. Essential oils like eucalyptus can help clear mucus and assist breathing pathways or even facilitate delivery of oxygen, etc. Many help inflammation, which can plague the body, or help bring relief which affects mood.

Patricia Davis, in Aromatherapy A-Z, says:

> *"Essential Oils can support and strengthen the immune response in two ways: by directly opposing the threatening microorganism or by stimulating and increasing the activity of the cells involved. A number of essential oils combine both these actions; for example,*

Lavender, Bergamot, Eucalyptus and Rosemary all act against a wide variety of bacteria and viruses while at the same time increasing the immune response. Rosemary and Geranium support the adrenal glands in their action and are also stimulants of the lymphatic system. Black Pepper and Lavender have a beneficial action on the spleen." (5)

A leading researcher in brain chemistry named Candace Pert says "your mind is in every cell of your body." (6) She discovered the opiate receptors and other peptide receptors in the brain and body, forming a continuous circuit with receptors in the brain, immune system, nervous system, hormonal system. "In other words, it is impossible to physiologically separate the mind from the body." (7). The mind-body connection is now a proven scientific fact

OUR BODY (NOSE & SCENT) WORKING WITH THE MIND AND SPIRIT

Did you know that we are capable of distinguishing millions of scents? While for a long time it was thought we could distinguish about 10,000 aromas, a study done in the eminent magazine Nature found that we actually detect millions! (8)

With the help of the olfactory nerves located in our nose, scents we inhale travel up to the area of the brain that controls our moods through the limbic system and onward from there.

Research by the Sense of Smell Institute reveals that while people's visual recall of images drops to about 50 percent after three months, they recall smells with a 65 percent accuracy after an entire year. (9)

Dr Mercola writes about the sense of scent (10):
Olfaction – the act of smelling – is especially geared for associative learning (in your hippocampus) and emotional processing (in your amygdala). Kate Fox explains it well in "The Smell Report":

> "Our olfactory receptors are directly connected to the limbic system, the most ancient and primitive part of the brain, which is thought to be the seat of emotion. Smell sensations are

relayed to the cortex, where 'cognitive' recognition occurs, only after the deepest parts of our brains have been stimulated. Thus, by the time we correctly name a particular scent as, for example, 'vanilla,' the scent has already activated the limbic system, triggering more deep-seated emotional responses."

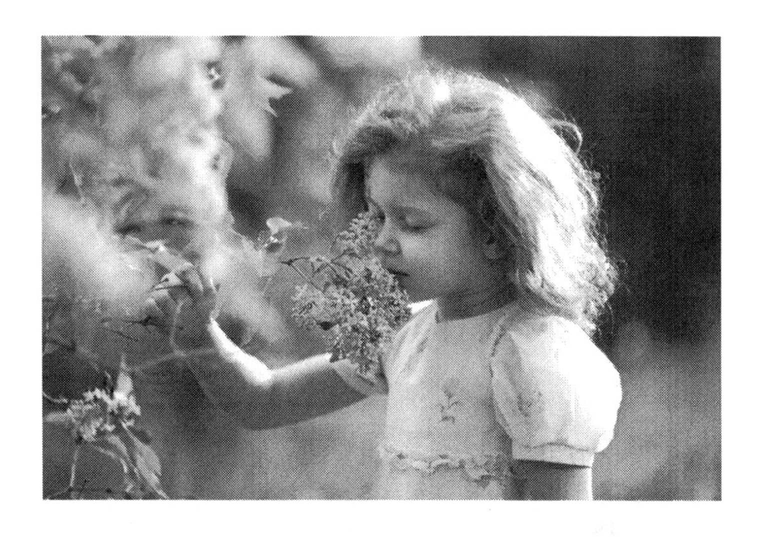

A number of studies have shown that odor learning begins before birth. A fetus detects flavor/odor compounds in its amniotic fluid, from the mother's diet. In studies where a mothers' consumption of distinctive smelling substances such as garlic, alcohol, or cigarette smoke were monitored during pregnancy, their infants were found to prefer these scents more than infants who had not been exposed to them.

After birth, newborns locate their mothers' nipples by smell. Breastfeeding also influences scent preferences; babies will associate breastfeeding smells with maternal bonding and the comfort of their mothers' arms. According to a recent study, babies can even smell their mothers' fears and learn the dangers of the world, just days after birth. When mothers experience stress, their body releases a scent that their baby detects and responds to.

Scent preferences change along with developmental stages. Studies show that three-year-olds have essentially the same likes and dislikes as adults. Children do not develop sensitivity to certain odors until they reach puberty. Researchers have also found that olfactory receptors differ by as much as 30 percent between any two individuals. On tests

> of smelling ability, women consistently score higher than men, and this gender difference holds true even for newborns!
>
> In summary, your responses to scents are largely "learned" as a function of the emotional context in which they were first experienced, and then the association influences your mood and behavior later in life. Naturally, there are genetic differences as well. Do you LOVE the smell of cilantro—or do you think it smells like soap? If the latter is true, you may be an olfactory mutant... literally. (10)

As aromatherapy's whole activity is olfaction, use of essential oils to help bolster wellness is amazing for our mind, body and spirit!

EPIGENETICS

As mentioned earlier in this chapter, another new area of study is epigenetics. As Dr. Mercola wrote, epigenetics reveal that you are an extension of your environment, which includes everything from your thoughts and belief systems, to toxic exposures and exposure to sunlight, exercise, and, of course, everything you choose to put onto and into your body. Epigenetics shatters the idea that you are a victim of your genes, and shows that you have tremendous power to shape and direct your physical health.

Our DNA has a coating called Epigenome that acts like a switch to turn off or on specific genes. While it was thought DNA was never changed, through Epigenetics, scientists now have information how these switches impact our health and the health of our children. (11)

EPIGENETICS AND ESSENTIAL OILS

Dr. Joshua Plant is a graduate of Harvard Medical School with a Ph.D. in biomedical sciences and Director of research at AMEO (Zija International). He and his team have conducted a massive experiment with essential oils to discover how they impact the genome – which genes essential oils may "turn on" or "turn off".

This experiment was exceptionally large, comprising over 40 different essential oils across 25,000 genes, with thousands of data points for each gene, ultimately yielding a database of literally billions of points of data on how essential oils impact human epigenetics.

As Améo's press office writes, this experiment, the first of its kind in the essential oil space, has spawned an immense amount of knowledge on how essential oils work on the human body. The science of essential oils has quickly evolved from understanding what comprises the essential oil, to understanding how essential oils impact the body... (12)

The database created by Dr. Plant "gives revolutionary insights into the influence essential oils have on our health, validating that which people have been experiencing from essential oils through trial and error for thousands of years. In addition to validating the efficacy of essential oils, it gives an unprecedented insight into how one can synergetically combine essential oils on an epigenetic scale to create a revolutionary insight of their true potential." (13)

One outcome of the Améo database is that while essential oils have traditionally been classified and categorized by their constituents (as we touch on in Chapter 7 and as mentioned in Chapter 1), these new studies classify them by their common theme of genes and what they do in specific systems.

6 zones were identified, and essential oils noted in each zone based on the tests of how they affected genes (14):

ZONE 1 – CIRCULATORY & RESPIRATORY

examples cinnamon, Eucalyptus globulus, and sandalwood

ZONE 2 – DIGESTIVE & EXCRETORY

examples frankincense, lavender, Eucalyptus radiata

ZONE 3 – LYMPHATIC & ENDROCRINE

examples lemon and Roman chamomile

ZONE 4 – MUSCULAR & REPRODUCTIVE

examples Clove and orange

ZONE 5- IMMUNE & NERVOUS

examples vetiver and grapefruit

ZONE 6 – SKELETON & INTEGUMENTARY

examples Bergamot, helichrysum, peppermint,

INVISIBLE FORCES

The mind, thoughts and emotions are invisible forces. Meditation and focus are invisible to us. What happens within the cell is invisible to the naked eye, as is what happens in our body when essential oils interact.

"Invisible forces are a fact of life. The air is full of invisible messages – from mobile phone conversations to satellite TV pictures. No biologist discusses physiological processes without talking about electricity, which you or I don't see. Physicists tell us that all life is basically vibration... Preliminary studies are proving what aromatherapists have long known – that essential oils have an effect far beyond the physical body." (15)

QUANTUM PHYSICS

Let's go beyond the physical body. Dr. David Stewart explores essential oils, the energy they hold and quantum physics. These concepts may be new to many and sound foreign, but keep an open mind.

Classic physics, as first developed by Sir Isaac Newton, deals with thing large enough to measure or see and experience with our senses. It deals with dimensions the size of an atom or larger.

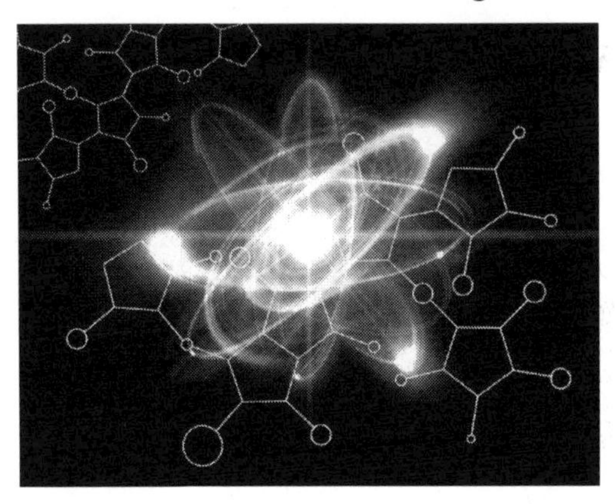

Quantum physic theories were first developed in the late 19th century and early 20th. explains the nature and behavior of matter and energy on the atomic and subatomic level, things too small to measure or see with our five senses. This includes energy.

"We know that the human mind can affect the electro-magnetic frequencies of essential oils. Prayer and positive thinking elevates frequencies while negative thoughts decrease the frequencies," writes Stewart. (16) He continues:

In the 1950's, an American scientist Franklin Loehr, explored the effect of human though and prayer on water. He discovered that human thought altered the bonding angles of oxygen and hydrogen atoms and changed the physical properties.

A Japanese scientist proved that human thought and emotion affected crystalline structures of frozen water. When beautiful thoughts with worlds like love, appreciation or angel were directed towards the ice, beautiful patterns were created. When negative thoughts with words like ugly, kill or demon were aimed at the ice, ugly crystals were formed.

The point being that thought, intent and emotion effect electron behavior. The so-called Mind-Body connection is through electrons.

We know that essential oils amplify intent – intent of the person using, inhaling or applying the oils (including a healing practitioner.)

Essential oils have electrical properties and are subject to our thoughts and emotions. In other words, the oil can do for you and your body what you need.

The compounds and constituents in the essential oil are the "packet of probabilities" offered by classic chemistry. Quantum physics is subject to the feeling, desire, emotion or intent, and can affect what the constituents present in the essential oil can accomplish.

Therapeutic grade essential oils are in a category all of the own – above and beyond the simple drugs, antibiotics and antibacterial agents.

Chemistry determines WHAT is possible; Quantum physics determines WHICH possibilities actually happen. Thoughts will not change the chemistry or compounds of an essential oil, but our thoughts can determine which will work or are needed. (16)

In addition to the various powers of essential oils discussed in the book, including the anti-microbial powers, immune system support, antioxidant powers, emotional aid (helping with sleep, stress, joy, pain, etc.) through the limbic system, Dr. Stewart suggests we add another super power: essential oil's ability to elevate frequencies in our body to stay well.

Chapter 7

MAGIC OF EXTRACTION… AND "CONSTITUENTS" THAT DEFINE THEIR POWER

"The best and safest thing is to keep a balance in your life, acknowledge the great powers around us and in us. If you can do that, and live that way, you are really a wise man." ~Euripides

We have explained that essential oils are the life force liquid found in plants. They are extracted from different parts of plants. This can be from the flower (such as lavender or chamomile), the grass (such as with lemongrass or palmarosa), the leaves (such as with cinnamon or peppermint), the peel (with lemon or bergamot), the stem or twig (such as with tea tree, eucalyptus or cypress), the seed (like cardamom) or wood (like cedarwood or rosewood).

The essential oil is extracted from the plant on different ways, depending on the plant.

Extraction is the process used to remove oil molecules from plant material. It's important to understand extraction because it determines an essential oil's properties, its benefits, how it's purchased and ways it is used.

The three primary methods of extracting essential oils are steam or water distillation, solvent extraction and expression (cold-pressing).

DISTILLATION BY STEAM

Distillation by steam under pressure is the most efficient means of extraction. Plant material is heated, a vapor forms and when it cools the resulting liquid is essential oil. In water distillation, plant material is covered in water and heated in a sealed container; this method takes longer than steam pressure and risks damaging delicate components of essential oils from longer exposure to heat. Steam distillation is the preferred and most commonly used method of extraction.

SOLVENT EXTRACTION

Solvent extraction is used for delicate petals such as jasmine and rose with a low yield of essential oil. This extraction is the end process of a method called "enfleurage", where petals are placed on glass and covered with an odorless fat or oil. An alternate method is to stir flowers into heated oil. Flowers are added until the oil or fat becomes saturated with flower essence, forming a substance called 'concrete' or 'pomade.' The pomade is soaked in alcohol which absorbs the fragrance of the fat, and the two are separated. The alcohol is allowed to evaporate, leaving particulate plant matter, the 'absolute' essence of the flower. The fat is used in soap manufacturing. When a synthetic petrochemical such as hexane or benzene is used as the solvent, the aromatherapy benefits of the absolute are inferior to those obtained with alcohol solvent, an organic substance derived from sugar or starch.

EXPRESSION

Expression (similar to cold-pressing or squeezing) is the method for extracting oil typically for citrus – always from the rind.

Bergamot, lemon, tangerine and orange are primary examples. Traditionally, this was a time consuming project done by hand; today, expression is mechanized. You may experiment with hand expression by cutting off a segment of peel from a washed and dried piece of fruit. Pierce the peel with your fingernail, or knife tip, and over a bowl use your fingers to squeeze drops of essential oil from the rind!

A WORD ON CARBON DIOXIDE

A fourth, more recent method of extraction utilizes carbon dioxide (CO2) process at lower temperatures. This method produces highly fragrant aromas and some aromatherapists believe the process is preferable to solvent extraction and steam distillation at higher temperatures. The CO2 process, however, requires expensive equipment which makes these oils costlier, as well as rare and difficult to obtain. Opponents of this type of this process believe the temperature in CO2 extraction is not high enough to properly distill plant molecules and that essential oils processed this way should be reserved for non-therapeutic uses, such as soap, candles and room deodorizers.

HYDROSOLS

In the process of extracting essential oils, hydrosols are produced with some types of plants. Hydrosol -

also called hydrolat, floral or flower water - is the water or vapor by-product of distillation. They are used in such things as skin tonics.

ABSOLUTES

It is the substance extracted through enfleurage using a solvent. In enfleurage, the flower petals are layered in wax or an animal fat. The wax or far becomes saturated with the oil from the plant or petals over several days until saturated. This scented wax or fat is now called a pomade. The pomade is washed in ethyl alcohol, a solvent to draw the fragrant molecules to it. After the alcohol evaporates, the result is the Absolutes.

They differ from Essential Oils in that they have lower concentrations but stronger perfume – they are typically used in perfumeries. They are not considered therapeutic at the level of essential oils.

CONSTITUENTS OF ESSENTIAL OILS

The main constituents that make up essential oils help us to understand their strengths and best applications.

Now, as you have learned, the makeup and complexity of each essential oil is vast. "One scientist estimated that just to identify all of the compounds present in the essential oils known today would take a thousand years." (1)

A typical essential oil user may not be as interested in the science or the constituents of essential oils, preferring to be told which oils to use for what. However, it is indeed helpful to have a rudimentary understanding of constituents or categories.

The following are compounds found in different essential oils. When you study what constituents are in a specific EO and their percentages, you begin to learn how they can be used. This is helpful for blending as well (picking 2 or more EOs that may help with the problem at hand.)

Remember, essential oils are subdivided into two distinct groups of chemical groups - the hydrocarbons which are made up almost exclusively of terpenes (monoterpenes, sesquiterpenes, and diterpenes), and the oxygenated compounds which are mainly esters, aldehydes, ketones, alcohols, phenols, and oxides. In general, terpenes inhibit the accumulation of toxins and help flush them.

Let's look at each general group and what they generally do. (You should understand that there are different constituents within EACH category, like linalool, menthol or terpinen-4, but we won't go into that in this book.) Examples of some essential oils in each group are included:

Monoterpenes - have antiseptic, anti-inflammatory and healing properties. Most essential oils have monoterpenes. Can be airborne sanitizers, decongesting in nature, skin penetration enhancers. Some examples of oils higher in monoterpenes are bergamot, frankincense, juniper, lemon, tea tree and thyme.

Sesquiterpenes are anti-inflammatory, antispasmodic and anti-infectious; they can also have calming qualities. They are heavier (denser) oils that can live longer. Examples that are high in sesquiterpenese include cedarwood, German chamomile, helichrysum, myrrh, vetiver and ylang ylang.

Monoterpenols (an alcohol): Anti-infectious, immune stimulants over the long term, healing for the skin, emotional balance. Linalol is a monoterpenol, found in lavender and clary sage. Other examples of oils high in monoterpenols are basil, geranium, neroli, peppermint and tea tree.

Sesquiterpenols: Anti-inflammatory, antiseptic, cooling, grounding, supports terrain antibiotic. These oils can help balance mind, body and energy. A high percentage of sesquiterpenols are found in cedarwood, sandalwood, patchouli and vetiver. These are heavier oils and can live longer.

Phenols are a stimulant to body systems, highly anti-infectious, strong immune stimulant and best used in small quantities. They are strong bactericidices. Two top examples high in phenols are Clove and Thyme. Phenols must always be diluted.

Esters are anti-bacterial, anti-spasmodic, and anti-infectious and some are healing to the skin. Many are sedative. Some examples high in esters include bergamot, cardamom, geranium, clary sage, helichrysum, lavender, Siberian fir, ylang ylang and Roman chamomile.

Ethers: Powerful antispasmodic effect, carminative, anti-infectious. They tend to have strong aromas. Examples are anise, nutmeg and tarragon.

Ketones are mucolytic; they can have relaxing, pain-relieves and sedative properties. Many are anti-coagulant. Some ketones must be used with caution. Camphor is a common ketone. Examples of essential oils high in ketones are peppermint, rosemary, vetiver and spike lavender.

Aldehydes can also be used as an antifungal, anti-inflammatory, cooling and to calm nerves. Dilution is important. An examples is lemongrass. Very unstable and can oxidize more quickly. Lemongrass is high in aldehydes.

Oxides (specifically 1,8 cineole). These are strong for the respiratory system (especially as a decongestant), antiviral, mentally stimulating and analgesic. Essential oils high in oxides include eucalyptus, rosemary, cardamom, and German chamomile.

When you look at the scientific studies, or analysis reports such as the GC/MS (gas chromatography-mass spectrometry) testing of an essential oil, you can understand more about what the essential oil can do by understanding the information above and what constituents specifically do. (Gas chromatography–mass spectrometry is an analytical method to identify different substances in the essential oil.) Some essential oils will have high percentages in several of the categories above, while others will be very strong in just one.

As discussed in the previous chapter, new studies by Dr. Joshua Plant have revealed how essential oils work in the cells, and he has classified essential oils into zones rather than just the constituents as above.

Chapter 8

MY TOP 15 ESSENTIAL OILS, BENEFITS AND PROPERTIES

"Healing with the clean, pure, beautiful agents of nature is surely the one method of all which appeals to most of us"

~ Dr. Edward Bach, 1936

There are hundreds of essential oils that are wonderful and can be added to your collection, depending on your wellness needs, but I decided to cover my top 15.

These are among the most common for wellness and your daily needs. There are plenty of books, encyclopedias and websites with information on all essential oils. I didn't think the need existed to cover them all here. It was hard to pick though - I left out such favorites as Clary Sage, Siberian Pine Needle, Sweet Orange and Oregano and I included one that is not as commonly used today in the U.S., Turmeric!

On the profiles in this chapter, I include a little history and/or some anecdotes not mentioned earlier; their qualities and uses, and what the special powers are. Thanks to Andrea Butje at Aromahead Institute, I also include some of the research she has pointed out.

My top 15 essential oils are:

Frankincense

Lavender

Rose Geranium

Eucalyptus

Peppermint

Clove Bud

Rosemary

Thyme

Myrrh

Lemon

Tea Tree

Helichrysum

Ylang Ylang

Bergamot

Tumeric

Let's take a look.

Frankincense (Boswellia carterii)

Frankincense is a tall shrub with papery bark

Countries of origin: Somalia, North Africa, Oman, India
Extraction Method: steam distillation
Plant part used: resin | gum
Also known as Olibanum; sometimes called "the King of Oils".

Some of the super powers of Frankincense:

- ✓ Mood**:** Frankincense is known for several for bringing tranquility, calm and focus while being uplifting (great for diffusing).
- ✓ Skincare**:** It is fantastic for skin (especially aging skin) as it helps regeneration, rejuvenation, oxygenation (it's an antioxidant) and in healing. It helps keeps tissues healthy. Add to your organic cream or oil for the face and body.
- ✓ Anti-Inflammatory Study: In the U.K., Cardiff University scientists found that Frankincense could inhibit the production of key inflammatory molecules, helping prevent the breakdown of the cartilage tissue that causes these conditions. (ScienceDaily August 4, 2011.) Put in your cream or oil, and massage on joints or affected areas twice daily.
- ✓ Respiratory Aid: Frankincense has good respiratory condition relief (use in an oil or cream on the chest, or in a bath)

- ✓ Bite, Cuts: Use Frankincense on an insect bite or in help healing cuts or wounds.
- ✓ Immune System: Frankincense supports your immune system and enhances health and wellness (as well as mood)! Could help oxygenate.
- ✓ Tonic**:** Frankincense oil is considered a tonic, as it benefits all the systems operating in the body, including the digestive, respiratory, nervous, and excretory systems.

Historical Anecdotes from the History Channel:

The ancient Egyptians bought entire boatloads of Frankincense and Myrrh from the Phoenicians: they used it for incense and burning, medicinal compounds for wounds, for insect repellent, in perfume and for their infamous embalming process. Frankincense was charred and ground into a power to make the heavy kohl eyeliner.

According to the Hebrew Bible, Frankincense and myrrh were components of the holy incense ritually burned in Jerusalem's sacred temples during ancient times.

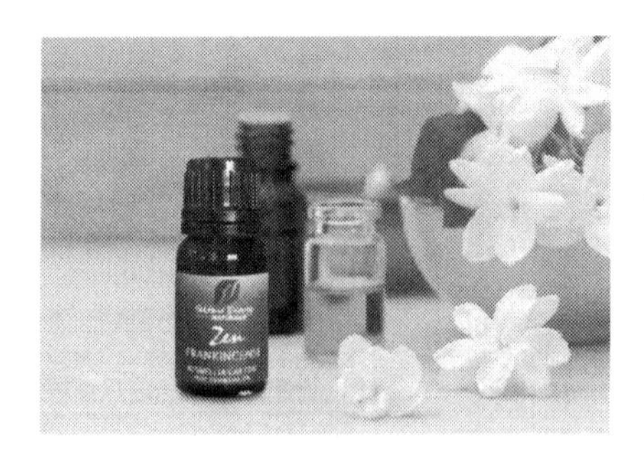

Peppermint (Mentha piperita)

Peppermint is an herb plant with lance shaped leaves.

Countries of origin: France, USA, Australia, India
Extraction Method: steam distillation
Plant part used: leaves

Peppermint plant is a hybrid of watermint and spearmint and was first described by Carl Linneaus in 1753. It's high menthol content distinguishes a top quality of Peppermint. Menthol is a well-known topical analgesic. It has the power to create a cooling and numbing sensation on the skin when low concentrations are applied, because ion channels are activated – but warmth in higher concentrations!

Warning: Peppermint is quite strong – keep any dosage for children at a very low amount.

Some of the many powers of Peppermint:

- ✓ Digestive support: Peppermint is very useful for a range of digestive problems, such as spasm, nausea, colic, and irritable bowel. Put some drops in an oil or cream and rub on the belly! It blends well with Fennel, Lemon, and Ginger for abdominal application. It's great in cool compresses for nausea, headaches and travel sickness.
- ✓ Fatigue: Peppermint is energizing and stimulating, and useful for both mental and physical fatigue.

- ✓ Pain relief: Peppermint is useful for local applications for pain relief like in a compress or a cloth for a headache rather than full body applications (e.g. massage and baths) as it is powerful.
- ✓ Circulation: Peppermint is known to help increase circulation in the area of application.
- ✓ Respiratory congestion: Peppermint can be inhaled on its own, or blended to reduce congestion.
- ✓ Antibacterial of course! It's an excellent antibacterial and antiviral.
- ✓ Liver and Immune System: It is known to support the liver.
- ✓ Pests: Rats, mice and insects apparently hate the smell of Peppermint.
- ✓ Oral Health. Peppermint has been used in mouthwashes or a drop in a toothpaste; it acts against specific bacteria.
- ✓ Mood: Peppermint is known to be energizing and refreshing as well as revitalizing. It can help ease the mind and bring focus.

Historical Anecdotes: In ancient Egypt, Peppermint was buried with the deceased to protect them on their journey into the afterlife.

A Greek myth says that Pluto loved a nymph named Minthe, but Pluto's wife grew so jealous that she turned Minthe into a plant. Pluto felt so bad about this that he bestowed on her a most pleasant scent later described as mint. (Small consolation, I say!)

The Ancient Greeks believed that misfortune was brought to those who rooted out or pulled up a mint plant. They were used under pillows at night for good dreams.

The Medieval French believed that carrying peppermint with St. John's Wort could scare off evil spirits.

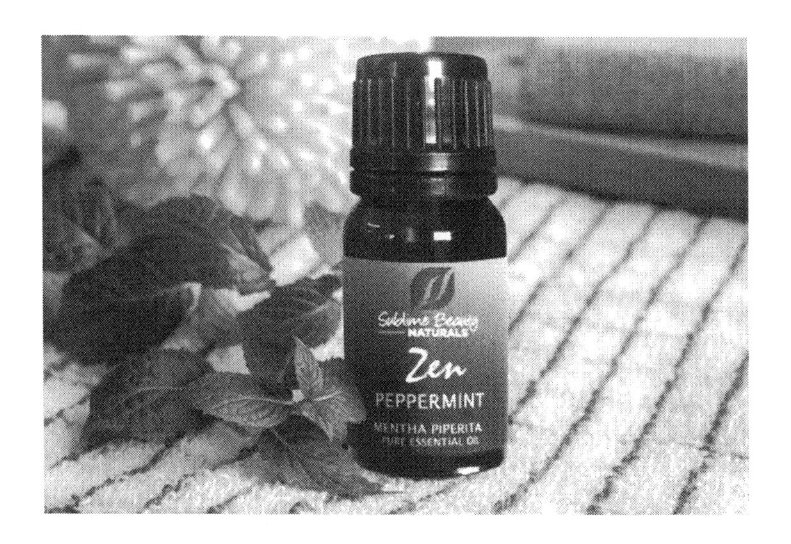

Lavender (Lavandula anguistifolia)

Lavender is a shrub with purple flowers.

Countries of origin: India, South of France, Italy, Bulgaria
Extraction Method: steam distillation
Plant part used: flowers

Some of the special powers from Lavender Essential Oil:

- ✓ Sleep, Stress or Anxiety: Lavender is well known for its outstanding sedative action on the nervous system, and for helping calm. It can be used for relaxation of tight muscles, tension headaches, spasmodic coughs and cramps. It blends well with Clary Sage or Bergamot for these actions.
- ✓ Anti-inflammatory and De-Stress: Related to stress and anxiety, Lavender is an excellent tonic for inflammation and physical pain.
- ✓ Cuts and Burns: Lavender is well-known to help heal cuts and burns. It brings a wonderful anti-bacterial power to play as well.
- ✓ Immune support: Lavender works well in blends to enhance immune function.
- ✓ Skin: Lavender can be combined with German Chamomile for allergies; with Tea Tree and/or Thyme ct. linalol for infections (including fungal infections and candida); and with Helichrysum and Geranium for trauma and healing.

- ✓ Analgesic: Lavender is well regarded as analgesic oil - its main constituent linalol has been well researched in this capacity.
- ✓ Antifungal: Lavender shows a good synergy with Tea Tree for healing athlete's foot. Lavender is also active against Candida.
- ✓ Antibacterial: Researchers at Cornell University have found lavender oil can eradicate certain antibiotic-resistant bacteria, including more than one strain of pathogenic Staphylococcus and pathogenic Streptococcus often involved in coughs and colds. Edwards-Jones et al. (2004) found that a combination of Lavender, Geranium, and Tea Tree had an increased inhibitory effect on the growth of methicillin-resistant Staphylococcus aureus (MRSA), but that Lavender and Tea Tree without the Geranium were less active against MRSA.
- ✓ Tonic: Lavender is considered an excellent tonic. It is healing on both body and mind, and can strengthen and restore vitality.

Historical Anecdotes: In 14th & 15th century Europe, Lavender tucked under the pillow of a young man was thought to encourage him to ask for his lady's hand in marriage. And Lavender was used by wives to ensure their "husband's marital passion."

Charles VI of France (1368-1422) demanded that his pillow always contain lavender so he could get a good night's sleep

Geranium or Rose Geranium (Pelargonium graveolens or Pelargonium asperum)
This is a beautiful scented flowering plant
Countries of origin: Egypt, China, Ile de Reunion, South Africa
Extraction Method: steam distillation
Plant part used: leaves

Note: The majority of aromatic geraniums (pelargoniums) are derived from two species, Pelargonium crispum and Pelargonium graveolens, which can also be referred to as Pelargonium asperum.

Some of the special powers of Rose Geranium:

- ✓ Uplifting Mood: Geranium is uniquely uplifting and anxiety relieving, also help with grief. It can be diffused or inhaled directly, or used in a cream. Great anti-depressant.
- ✓ Lymphatic Support: Geranium has a gentle stimulating effect on the lymphatic system. It can be very useful for reducing edema and fluid retention. For swollen ankles, Geranium can be used in a bath, blended into a cream or oil, or added to a cool foot soak.
- ✓ Analgesic and Post-Shingles: It can rapidly relieve the pain of post herpetic neuralgia, a complication from shingles that causes nerve pain. (1)
- ✓ Anti-inflammatory and anti-bacteria: Like most essential oils, Rose Geranium is a great anti-

bacterial agent and thanks to its constituents, a good anti-inflammatory as well. As mentioned earlier in the book, Edward-Jones et al. (2) investigated the effects of the vapors (in vitro) from several oils, including Geranium (alone and in combination), on Staphylococcus aureus, MRSA, and epidemic methicillin-resistant S. aureus (EMSRA). Geranium oil showed excellent inhibition, and Geranium combined with Tea Tree was the most active against MRSA.

- ✓ Skin care: Geranium is wonderful for skin and hair care. It balances sebum and help with excess oil or dryness.

Historical Anecdote: The Zulus and the Hottentots of South Africa have a long history of using Pelargonium graveolens for medicinal purposes

Comment on its therapeutic qualities: Interestingly, Dr. Kurt Schnaubelt notes about Rose Geranium oil: "The tonifying effect of the terpene alcohol combined with the soothing influence of the esters are responsible for the fact that geranium is perceived differently for each individual. One person will perceive it as antiseptic, another as calmative, and a third as stimulant...because of this versatile character, geranium is an excellent foundation for massage and body oils.

Eucalyptus (Eucalyptus globulus)

Eucalyptus is a very tall tree with blue-green leaves.

Countries of origin: Originally native to Australia; Spain, China, Portugal

Extraction Method: steam distilled

Plant part used: leaves.

Some of the powers of Eucalyptus:

- ✓ Respiratory and Sinus Support: Eucalyptus is a decongestant, an expectorant and mycolytic. It is a top essential oil for helping the respiratory system, containing about 70% eucalyptol.
- ✓ Antibacterial: Eucalyptus essential oil is effective against a range of bacterial respiratory pathogens and is excellent to fight respiratory and airborne bacteria.
- ✓ Antifungal: The essential oil is dominated by 1,8 cineole, which is active against Candida species (Kordali et al. 2005) and other fungi.
- ✓ Antioxidant: The essential oil has demonstrated good antioxidant activity
- ✓ Astringent: The essential oil can decrease sebum production as it can reduce the size of sebaceous glands (Bhatt et al. 2011).
- ✓ Immune Support: It is believed that Eucalyptus has an immunostimulant capacity, possibly on account of its antimicrobial, anti-inflammatory, and tonic actions.
- ✓ Increases cerebral blood flow: Inhalation of 1,8 cineole, the major constituent of Eucalyptus oil,

increases cerebral blood flow (3) This can help with mental fatigue.

- ✓ Restores Positive Energy: Eucalyptus helps dispel depression and brings positivity. It cleans and refreshes the spirit.

Historical Tidbits: In 1855, the French government sent Eucalyptus seeds to Algeria and many fever zones with malaria. The disease-ridden areas were converted to healthy dry areas that became malaria-free. This was actually thanks to the German botanist Baron Ferdin and Von Muller's suggestion that using Eucalyptus plants could prove to be antiseptic. As early as the 1880s, surgeons were already using eucalyptus oil as an antiseptic during operations

Eucalyptus was in demand during World War I as it helped control a meningitis outbreak and was used for the influenza of 1919.

Warnings: Be careful with children under ten years of age. Also, take care if you are asthmatic. Although research shows it can be helpful with bronchial asthma, it also shows concern that it might set off an asthma attack in certain cases.

Clove Bud (Eugenia caryophyllata)
Clove is an evergreen tree with dark green leaves and pink flowers
Countries of origin: Indonesia, Zanzibar, Madagascar
Extraction Method: steam distilled
Plant part used: Closed buds of the flowers.

Some of the special powers of Clove Bud:

- ✓ Strong Anti-bacterial and Anti-fungal**:** Clove is a strong bactericide! It is one of three essential oils in which no bacteria, virus or fungi can live in its presence. Clove has a wide spectrum of antimicrobial activities that is well tested and used. When combined with Rosemary and Lavender, it has additive effects against Gram positive and Gram negative bacteria. (4) Tests demonstrated that Clove Bud essential oil has activity against HSV I and HSV II. (5)
- ✓ Anti-inflammatory and Analgesic: Clove Bud is dominated by eugenol, which has excellent anti-inflammatory action and pain relief abilities.
- ✓ Immune System Support: Clove Bud essential oil can stimulate the immune system.
- ✓ Anti-coagulant**:** Eugenol and Clove Bud have anti-platelet aggregation actions. Useful to clot blood, but caution if you are prone to blood clots.
- ✓ Anti-depressant: Monoamine oxidase (MAO) is an enzyme that breaks down serotonin,

dopamine, adrenalin, and noradrenalin. Eugenol is thought to inhibit MAO, hence has potential antidepressant actions (but don't use if on MAO inhibiting drugs.)

- ✓ Digestive Problems: Clove is wonderful digestive oil, and has been used for millennia for this purpose. It can be added to blends that are massaged into the abdomen to assist digestion.
- ✓ Warming: Clove offers warming effects and is strengthening for the body overall. Clove Bud can be used sparingly in massage blends and creams for pain and discomfort due to inflammation, and for nerve pain such as sciatica. It has a warming effect on the senses. It can be incorporated in an inhaler blend, or a massage blend with Rose, Orange, Geranium, or Ylang Ylang.. Clove Bud can be used sparingly in massage blends and creams for pain and discomfort due to inflammation, and for nerve pain such as sciatica. It has a warming effect on the senses. It can be incorporated in an inhaler blend, or a massage blend with Rose, Orange, Geranium, or Ylang Ylang.

Warning: May cause skin and mucous membrane irritation or sensitization – Always dilulte it. Limit topical use to maximum of 0.5%. Avoid using with children. Avoid using on any sensitive or damaged skin. Eugenol (Clove) is a potent prostaglandin inhibitor, and is to be avoided by people with significant renal (kidney) disease.

Historical Anecdote: Gattefossé mentioned a report from J. Cloquet that when the Dutch destroyed the clove trees rampant on the Island of Ternate (in the Moluccas archipelago), the colony was decimated by several epidemics diseases never before seen. It was believed that the power of the clove leaves and flowers were able to purify the air to prevent the diseases (and they were probably right.)

Anecdote 2: In 1522, Magellan's ship returned from its fateful trip around the world loaded with Clove, to the delight of Spain. (Magellan himself was killed in the Philippines).

Anecdote 3: The Chinese have used Clove for well over 2000 years. In the west, using clove for toothaches was first documented in the French "Practice of Physic" in 1640.

WARNINGS: May cause skin and mucous membrane irritation or sensitization. Limit topical use to maximum of 0.5% dilution. Avoid using Clove with children. Avoid using on any sensitive or damaged skin. Eugenol (Clove) is to be avoided by people with significant renal (kidney) disease or liver disease.

Lemon (citrus limon)

The lemon tree is an evergreen with yellow lemon fruit
Countries of Origin: Spain, Italy, France, S. Africa
Plant Part Used: Fresh Fruit Rind
Extraction Method: Cold Pressed.

Some of the powers of Lemon essential oil:

- ✓ Antiseptic and anti-bacterial**:** Dr. Valnet wrote that "The essence of lemon is second to none in its antiseptic and bactericidal properties. The works of Morel and Rochaiz have demonstrated that the vapors of lemon essence alone will neutralize the meningococcus in 15 minutes, the typhus bacillus in less than an hour, pneumonococcus in one to three hours, staphylococcus in two hours and hemolytic streptococcus in three to 12 hours. Applied directly, the essential oil itself neutralizes the typhus bacillus and staphylococcus in only five minutes and the diphtheria bacillus in just 20 minutes." (6) Lemon is great to diffuse if there are sick ones in the house to purify the air and add freshness.
- ✓ Immune System Aid**:** With its antibacterial and antioxidant actions, anti-inflammatory actions, and activating, tonic effects on the mind and body, Lemon essential oil can be used to help support the immune system and promote well-being.

- ✓ Liver support/protector: d-Limonene can increase the rate of synthesis of glutathione S-transferase in the liver. This is an important enzyme in detoxification pathways (7)
- ✓ Analgesic and anti-inflammatory: Can reduce the sensation of pain, thanks to the main component, d-limonene, a good anti-inflammatory. Also cooling activity. Blend with Frankincense, Ginger, Lavender, Geranium or Juniper Berry to help counteract inflammation and pain.
- ✓ Antidepressant: Lemon essential oil can decrease both physical and psychological stress. It is good to diffuse to refresh and uplift mood.
- ✓ Antispasmodic: The antispasmodic actions of Lemon are likely due in part to the presence of d-limonene, a vaso-relaxant.
- ✓ Astringent: Many citrus oils, including Lemon and those containing high levels of monoterpenes (such as limonene), can contract and tighten the tissues. It can be a good skincare tonic and is also useful for oily skin when blended with a carrier.
- ✓ Diuretic: When used in a blend, Lemon can contribute to a diuretic effect.
- ✓ Circulation: Lemon can help reduce swelling and pain associated with varicose veins, especially if combined with Cypress and Patchouli. It can help increase circulation.

- ✓ Nausea**:** Lemon is helpful for reducing nausea, especially when combined with Peppermint.
- ✓ Overall Well-Being: Because Lemon is an immune system stimulant, and protects and nourishes the liver, and is a great bactericide, it is a great one to diffuse. It is fresh. Also a great essential oil to use in household cleaning products to disinfect and purify while freshening. It is also good for reducing nausea, especially when combined with Peppermint.

Warning: Like all citrus essential oils, lemon be photo-toxic (take care if applying topically followed by time in the sun.)

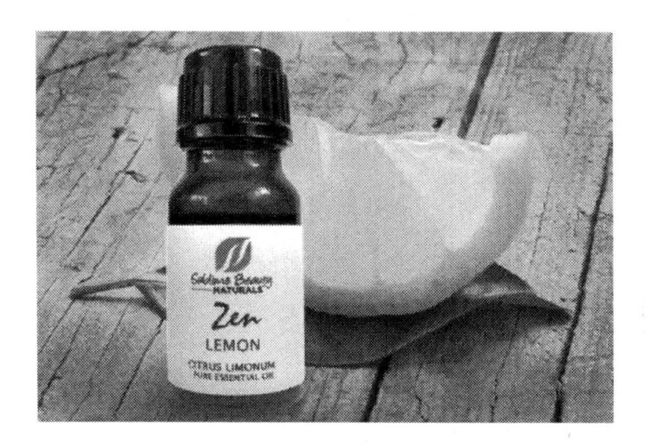

Rosemary (Rosemarinus officinalis)

Rosemary is a hardy evergreen shrub

Countries of Origin: Spain, France, S. Africa
Extraction Method: Steam Distilled
Plant Part Used: Leaves, Twigs.

Some of the powers of Rosemary essential oil:

- ✓ Stimulation: Massage with Rosemary oil can increase attentiveness, alertness, liveliness, and joyfulness, while increasing breathing rate and blood pressure (8) Rosemary can promote alertness and cognitive performance, shown following clinical tests. (9) Could help with long-term memory.
- ✓ Stress and Cortisol: Directly related to stimulation, Rosemary has been shown in many tests to bring down Cortisol levels, which are high during stress. Using it can help with stress symptoms including fatigue and depression.
- ✓ Analgesic and Anti-Inflammatory: Rosemary (which includes camphor as a constituent) can reduce inflammation and pain. Can be used to reduce headaches. Early herbalists like Culpeper have recommended Rosemary for numb joints.
- ✓ Antibacterial and Antifungal**:** Numerous tests have shown Rosemary to have wide
- ✓ antibacterial powers, like most essential oils. In addition, clinical tests show it synergistic with Clove against Candida albicans (10)

- ✓ Respiratory aid: Rosemary helps with respiration, and also helps with congestion and coughs, getting mucus out. Blend some in a cream, mix with Lavender, Eucalyptus and Frankincense for synergy and aid.
- ✓ Circulatory stimulant: Rosemary also has a long-standing reputation for increasing circulation and is often added to blends for this purpose.
- ✓ Fighting Mental Fatigue: Rosemary ct. 1,8 cineole can be diffused or inhaled to help increase alertness and alleviate mental fatigue. In ancient Rome, it was known as a "happiness" plant.
- ✓ Mood: Rosemary is known for helping with enthusiasm, inspiration, creativity, memory and strengthening of spirit.

Historical Anecdote: In Hamlet, Shakespeare wrote Ophelia to say 'There's rosemary - that's for remembrance'. One of the powers of Rosemary is enabling of memory and alertness, proven by modern clinical researchers.

Warnings: Epilepsy - Robert Tisserand suggests avoiding rosemary-chemotype-camphor at levels higher than 16%. Children - do not apply rosemary on or near the face of infants or children under 5 years old. Use with caution for children between 5-10 years old.

Thyme (Thymus vulgaris)

Thyme is a small low-growing herb with typically pinkish flowers

Countries of Origin: Spain, France, S. Africa
Plant Part Used: Flowers, Leaves.
Extraction Method: Steam Distilled

Some of the powers of Thyme essential oil:

- ✓ Antibacterial, Antifungal & Airborne Antimicrobial: Thyme oils are well regarded for their antiseptic vapors. Linalol (a main constitutent) has strong powers against many bacteria, fungi and viruses. It helps prevent infection, and helps to heal wounds. This is one of the essential oils proven to kill Staph. If suffering a viral infection, blend Thyme with Lemon and Clove Bud in a carrier – rub into chest and neck.
- ✓ Analgesic and Anti-inflammatory: The main constituents of Thyme (including linalol) give it analgesic and anti-inflammatory power. (Guimarães et al. 2013).
- ✓ Respiratory Relief**:** Thyme can alleviate coughs, congestion and spams. Dr. Balvay wrote in Paris 1921 that it helped relieve tuberculosis symptoms. To unblock passages, use 3 drops Thyme and 3 drops Peppermint.
- ✓ Antioxidant: Thyme essential oils have significant antioxidant activity (Wei and Shibamoto 2010). The component linalol also has antioxidant action.

- ✓ Antispasmodic: The essential oil has antispasmodic activity on gastrointestinal tract tissues (in vitro) (Meister et al. 1999).
- ✓ Calming Factor: Inhaled linalol can repress stress and contributes to anxiety relief. Topically, it also calms skin.
- ✓ Immune System: Thyme is believed to support the immune system; its antioxidant, antimicrobial, anti-inflammatory and stress relieving actions support this belief. It is gentle yet effective.
- ✓ Mood: Thyme helps sooth, calm and helps dissolve feelings of heaviness. It is a gentle and warming essential oil.

Historical Anecdote: The word Thyme comes from the Greek meaning to "fumigate". 2000 years ago in Greece, it was a mark of high respect to say someone smelled of thyme! It was used for purification in temples and homes, and was most revered.

According to legend, Thyme was born from the tears of Helen of Troy.

In Danish and German folklore, wild Thyme was a place where you would find fairies.

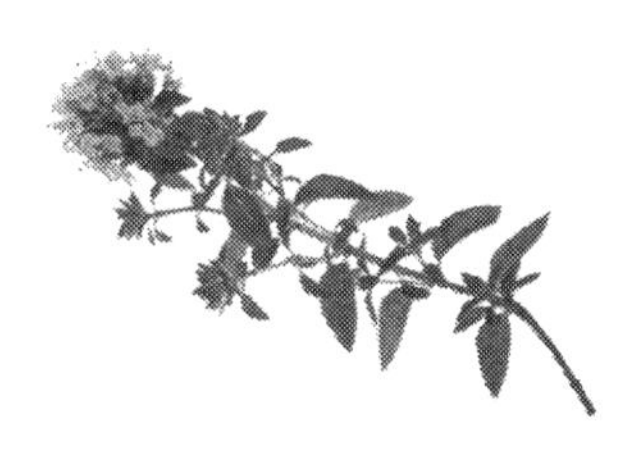

Tea Tree | Melaleuca (Melaleuca alternifolia)

Tea Tree is an evergreen

Countries of Origin: Native to Australia; S. Africa
Plant Part Used: Leaves.
Extraction Method: Steam Distilled

Note: Tea Tree is quite rich in terpinen-4-ol, a very effective antimicrobial.

Some of the powers of Tea Tree essential oil:

- ✓ Acne Treatment**:** Well-known and tested in the treatment of acne; it also helps reduce lesions.
- ✓ Anti-bacterial and Airborne Antimicrobial: The components, including terpinen-4-ol, α-terpineol, and α-pinene, are active against Staphylococcus aureus, S. epidermidis and Propionibacterium acnes (11), and MRSA, Candida and a wide spectrum of microbes. Tea Tree is well suited to diffuse as an aerial antiseptic. It was demonstrated (12) that the vapors of Tea Tree in conjunction with Geranium were the most active against MRSA of all the oils and combinations investigated.
- ✓ Anti-Fungal: Tea Tree is an exceptional product to fight fungus. It is active against dermatophytes, and against clinical Candida species (thanks to component 1,8 cineole). Tea Tree is shown to be synergistic with Clove as well.

- ✓ Oral Care: Tea Tree is known to aid in oral care. 1 drop in toothpaste daily can help prevent gum disease, infections including oral candidiasis, and prevent sore throats.
- ✓ Analgesic and Anti-inflammatory: Tea Tree can reduce pain and reduce inflammation.
- ✓ Allergies: Tea Tree and terpinen-4-ol can alleviate allergies by suppressing histamine release and cytokine production (13).
- ✓ Respiratory Problems: Tea Tree can help resolve or relieve respiratory problems, including those from allergies.
- ✓ Antiviral: Tea Tree oil has an inhibitory effect on a subtype of H1N1, and shows promise in the treatment of influenza. (14)
- ✓ Immune System: Tea Tree's powers —antimicrobial, antiviral, anti-inflammatory, and antiallergy—help support a strong immune system.
- ✓ Mood: Tea Tree helps refresh the mind, gives feelings of optimism and helps energize.

Anecdotes: Australian aborigines crush tea tree leaves for a poultice that treats skin infections, wounds, and burns. Melaleuca Alternifolia got the name Tea Tree from Captain James Cook, a lieutenant with the British Royal Navy, who used the leaves to brew tea.

Ylang Ylang (Cananga odorata)

Ylang Ylang is a tropical tree with large star-shaped flowers which are first produced in the 5th year of the tree's life.

Countries of Origin: Madagascar, Ile de Reunion, Comoro (native to the Philippines and Malaysia)

Plant Part Used: Flowers.

Extraction Method: Steam Distilled

Some powers of Ylang Ylang essential oil include:

- ✓ Antidepressant**:** The scent of Ylang Ylang is well known for its uplifting, euphoric effects which can counteract low mood or depression. It is a sensual, soothing and exotic scent which heightens feelings and helps with creativity, reducing stress. Excellent in a massage oil, or in a bath.
- ✓ Analgesic and Anti-inflammatory: Some of the components, including linalol, have pain relieving actions as well as good anti-inflammatory power. Helps relieve muscular tension, too.
- ✓ Calming and Hypertension: Ylang Ylang can help lower blood pressure and heart rate. (15) It can help relieve trauma. Inhalation of a blend of Ylang Ylang, Bergamot and Lavender reduced psychological stress responses (16)
- ✓ Skin healing: In some cultures, Ylang Ylang is used in skin care products, and is mixed with coconut oil for the treatment of skin problems

(17) Excellent for moisturizing agent blended in creams.

- ✓ Mood: Harmonizing, calming, eases the mind, helps if feeling withdrawn, helps heighten senses and brings joy.

Historical Anecdote: Ylang Ylang essential oil was used in the 19th century as a hair oil. In the Philippines, it was used as protection from snakebites and harsh saltwater, and in the healing of cuts and burns; the oil was mixed with coconut oil as the carrier.

In Indonesia, the petals of Ylang Ylang flowers are scattered over the bed of newlywed couples on their wedding night.

French chemists Garnier and Rechler, working on the Ile of Reunion in the early 20th century, first noticed the therapeutic powers of Ylang Ylang; they noticed it was an effective treatment for all types of diseases including malaria, typhus and intestinal infections. They also wrote of its calming effect on fast heartbeats.

Ylang Ylang essential oil is used as a floral top note in the ever-popular Chanel No. 5 perfume (my favorite perfume when I lived in Paris.)

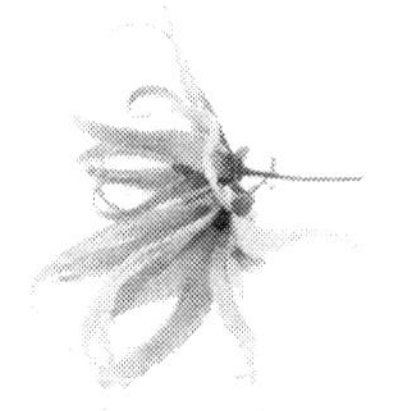

Myrrh (Commiphora myrrha)

Myrrh is a tough little shrubby tree with sharp needles.
Countries of Origin: Ethiopia, S. Africa
Plant Part Used: Resin/Gum.
Extraction Method: Steam Distilled

Some of the powers of Myrrh include:

- ✓ Mood: Similar to Frankincense, Myrrh can help ease the mind, dissolve anger and create a sense of tranquility and peace.
- ✓ Antibacterial: After the discovery of bacteria it was found that myrrh was an effective antibacterial agent killing Staphylococcus aureus and other gram-positive organisms.
- ✓ Analgesic and Anti-inflammatory powers: Myrrh has very good analgesic and anti-inflammatory powers. It is actually used in Chinese medicine for arthritis (18), and in Ayurveda for inflammatory diseases (19). It is warming and excellent in blends for arthritis, inflammation, muscular pain and overall pain. It blends well with Frankincense, Clove Bud, Juniper Berry and Black Pepper.
- ✓ Skin: Myrrh is known to help protect skin, and help slow-healing wounds and damages. It offers a regenerating power, along with anti-inflammatory and antioxidant powers. It could help with such conditions as eczema and athlete's foot (blended with Tea Tree). Further, it can help stop bleeding.

- ✓ Respiratory Aid: It has good powers to help decongest, and is often blended for calming coughs.
- ✓ Circulatory: Myrrh stimulates blood circulation and ensures the proper supply of oxygen to the tissues.
- ✓ Oral Care: Myrrh is an antiseptic and is most often used in mouthwashes, gargles and toothpastes for prevention and treatment of gum disease.
- ✓ Antispasmodic: Myrrh can help relieve spasms, cramps and contractions.
- ✓ Antioxidant: Myrrh essential oil is a singlet oxygen quencher. (20) In ancient Egypt, Myrrh was used in rejuvenating facial treatments (and medicinally).

Warnings: Contraindicated for pregnancy and breastfeeding

Historical Anecdotes: Myrrh, in its various forms has been used for as long as there is recorded history. It is mentioned in the oldest epic, the Gilgamesh from Mesopotamia.) We read the story in the history chapter about the ancient Egyptian war general Milkili, who refused to go to war without a supply of Myrrh from the Pharoah.

Myrrh is mentioned in so many ancient documents including in the clay tablets of Mesopotamia, in the Ebers Papyrus (we read about it in the history chapter) as a component of the classic medicine & compound Kyphi, in the writings of Greek and Roman authors, and in the Bible. It is the first essential oil mentioned in the Bible, in Genesis. Queen Esther, (Esther 2:12) was massaged with Myrrh for 6 months in preparation for her marriage to the king. Myrrh was offered by the Magi at the birth of Jesus.

In ancient Greece and Rome Myrrh was used as a remedy for skin sores, for treating mouth and eye infections, as a cough remedy, against worm infestation and for cattle abdominal pains. According to Touwaide, Myrrh appears with more frequency than any other plant substance in the writings of the Greek physician Hippocrates, who revolutionized the field of medicine in the fourth and third centuries B.C.

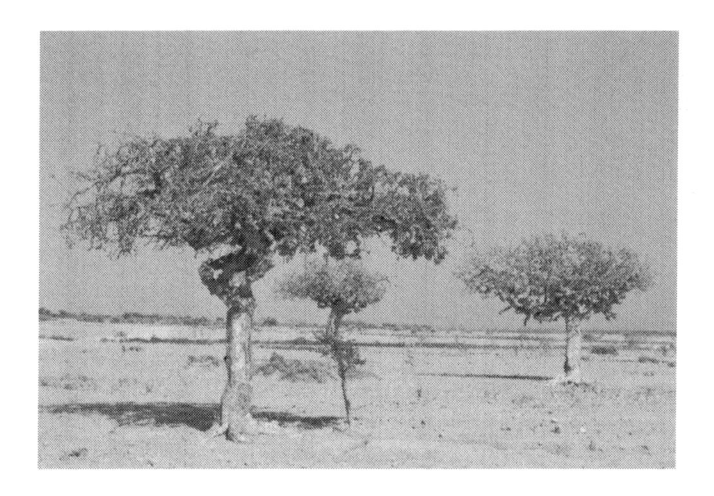

Helichrysum (Immortelle) (Helichrysum italicum)

Helichrysum (also called Everlasting) is an herb with grayish-green leaves and yellow flowers.

Countries of Origin: Corsica, Italy, USA, Bosnia, Croatia

Plant Part Used: Flowers. Helichrysum is an herb with grayish-green leaves and yellow flowers.

Extraction Method: Steam Distilled

Some of the powers of Helichrysum essential oil:

- ✓ Wound healing: A clinical test investigated the therapeutic effects and potential clinical applications of Helichrysum diluted in oil of musk rose (Rosa rubiginosa) after cosmetic and reconstructive surgery. This combination reduced inflammation, edema, and bruising. (21) It is now well-known that Helichrysum heals cuts. Put 1 drop neat on a fresh cut – it helps stop the bleeding and begins the healing process (as well as acting as an antibacterial). Follow with Lavender to aid the healing process, if desired.
- ✓ Prevents Bruising: Helichrysum has the ability to prevent and alleviate bruising after soft tissue trauma.
- ✓ Antibacterial: Helichrysum is like most essential oils – it acts as an antibacterial. It significantly reduced the multidrug resistance of the Enterobacter aerogenes, E.coli, Pseudomonas aeruginosa, and Acetobacter

baumanni. (22) Helichrysum was also included in a study investigating the antimicrobial activities of floral-aroma essential oils. All of the oils and most of the principal aroma compounds showed medium-to-high antimicrobial activities against both Gram-positive and Gram-negative bacteria. (23) Health Sciences Research Centre at the University of Beira in Portugal found that Helichrysum's constitutents - flavonoids and terpene - were effective against bacteria and fungus growth. (24)

- ✓ Analgesic and Anti-Inflammatory: Helichrysum has pain relieving and anti-inflammatory actions, probably thanks to a constituent neryl acetate.
- ✓ Heart Health: A study by the University of Durban (School of Medical Sciences) in South Africa, showed the hypotensive action of helichrysum improves the condition of blood vessels by lowering inflammation, increasing smooth muscle function and lowering high blood pressure. (25)
- ✓ Relieves Sunburn and Skin Allergies: By reducing inflammation, pain, and swelling, Helichrysum can be used to relieve allergies that manifest in the skin.
- ✓ Musculoskeletal: Helichrysum is very useful for muscle and tendon damage, inflammation, bruising, joint pain, and swelling. It can be blended for local application.

- ✓ Antidepressant: It acts as an antidepressant; excellent to diffuse or use in a massage oil.
- ✓ Liver Detox: According to Dr. Axe, Known to be an antispasmodic, blood purifier and anti-inflammatory, Helichrysum has been used as a liver stimulant and detoxifier for centuries. It's commonly used in folk medicine to treat liver disease and to help the body detoxify from toxins, heavy metals, bacteria and air pollution. (26)
- ✓ Mood: Uplifting, sweet, protective, helps bring inner calm, a sense of well-being and feelings of peace.

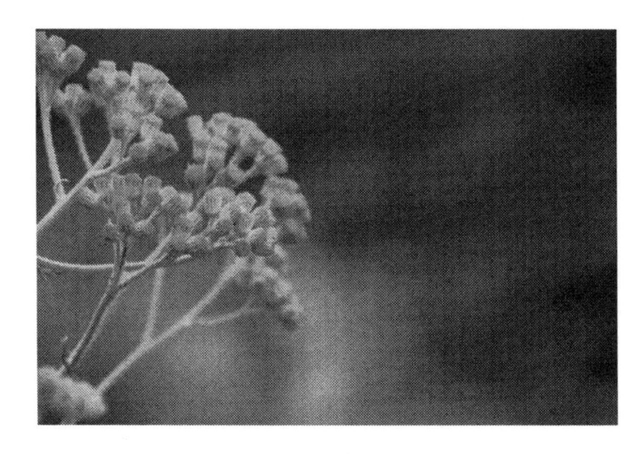

Bergamot (Citrus bergamia)

Bergamot is a small citrus tree, and the fruit has a green peel.

Countries of Origin: Italy and Brazil
Plant Part Used: Fresh Fruit Rind.
Extraction Method: Cold Pressed

Some of the special powers of Bergamot essential oil:

- ✓ Analgesic: Bergamot has analgesic power, and it's been established that both linalool and linalyl acetate (constituents found in Bergamot) have these powers. According to one study, it has potential in the treatment of cancer pain and related depression and anxiety (28)
- ✓ Anti-inflammatory: Often cited as having anti-inflammatory action thanks to the constituents linalool and d-limonene. It's a wonderful oil to help bring down inflammation.
- ✓ Antibacterial and Antifungal: Bergamot has long been used in folk medicine to treat infections; today it is found to fight microbes and fungi. In one in vitro study Bergamot worked against common dermatophytes (29) and was active in vitro against clinical Candida isolates in another study. (30) Active against a number of respiratory pathogens.
- ✓ Specific Antibiotic-Resistant Bacteria: The Journal of Applied Microbiology published that Bergamot oil can produce positive results against Enterococcus faecium and

Enterococcus faecalis bacteria, resistant to the potent antibiotic vancomycin. These enterococcal species are a common source of a variety of infections, including urinary tract infections (UTI), bacteremia, endocarditis, and meningitis. Just add bergamot oil to your sitz bath or hip bath to help prevent the spread of bacterial infections from the urethra into the bladder.(31)

- ✓ Antidepressant: When inhaled along with Ylang Ylang and Lavender, Bergamot reduced psychological stress responses and serum cortisol levels, and reduced the blood pressure of patients with essential hypertension. (32) In a hand massage blend with Lavender and Frankincense, Bergamot helped alleviate pain and depression in cancer patients (33)
- ✓ Respiratory Aid: Bergamot has antispasmodic powers, which can help calm a cough.
- ✓ Ease Flatulence: Bergamot mixed with Roman Chamomile and/or Peppermint in a massage oil – rub your tummy – can help with treatment of gas, indigestion, and flatulence.
- ✓ Restless Leg Syndrome and Muscle Tensions: Bergamot works in massage oils to reduce tension and soothe painfully tight muscles, and it helps with restless leg syndrome.
- ✓ Stress: Bergamot is useful for soothing depression, stress and anxiety. It blends well with other antidepressant oils such as

Geranium or Lavender. Diffuse it, or use in a massage oil blend.

- ✓ **Mood and Emotional Health**: Supports emotional health and well-being. Diffuse it alone or blend with Clary Sage or Rosemary. Bergamot can gently release pent-up emotions or anger, and it relieves feelings of apathy. Its mood is refreshing and nurturing and helps with feelings of positivity.

Warning: Like all citrus oils, Bergamot is phototoxic. Avoid direct sunlight or tanning beds for up to 18 hours after applying Bergamot to the skin; serious skin burn can occur. Bergamot must not be applied to the skin undiluted.

Historical Anecdote: An essence extracted from the aromatic skin of this sour fruit is used in Earl Grey and Lady Grey teas, and in the confectionery Turkish Delight. It is often found in marmalade in Europe (especially Italy).

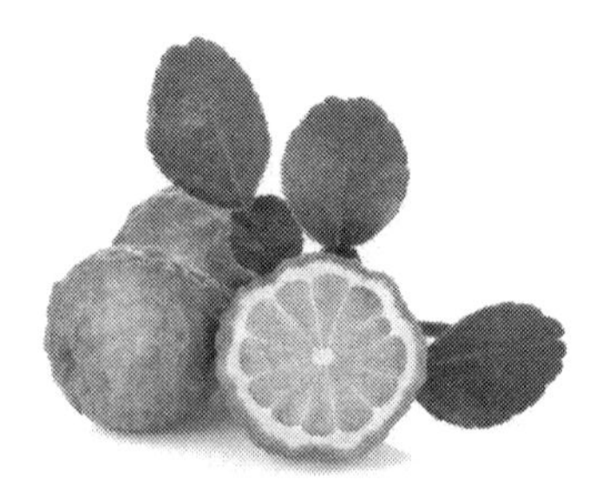

Turmeric (Curcuma longa)

This is a tropical plant with a fleshy bulbous root
Countries of Origin: India, Madagascar, China, Indonesia, Japan
Plant Part Used: Roots
Extraction Method: Steam distillation

Tumeric has been used extensively throughout history (less so now but it may be rediscovered in the west). In Ayurveda, it is used as an all-round internal cleansing tonic. In Chinese medicine, it is used for sores, bruises, chest pain, tooth ache and was once a cure for jaundice. High in vitamins and minerals, especially Vitamin C. Curcumin is extracted from turmeric, known as the Indian spice Curry. The essential oil has a deeper, root-like scent that is subtle and is related to ginger. It's not a "pretty" floral but quite medicinal!

Powers of turmeric essential oil:

- ✓ Anti-inflammatory and Analgesic: It's powerful to help bring down inflammation throughout the body. It helps control the extent of inflammation and acts as an analgesic. Known to aid in arthritis, muscular aches and rheumatism. A recent study out of Japan evaluated its relationship with interleukin (IL)-6, the inflammatory cytokine known to be involved in the RA process, and discovered that curcumin "significantly reduced" these inflammatory markers. (36) Put turmeric and bergamot in a bath or foot bath; blend in a massage oil or cream as well as inhale or diffuse.

- ✓ Antibacterial and Antifungal: Like most essential oils, it has the powers to kill microbes Clinical tests showed turmeric killed fungus more effectively than ginger, clove and oregano. (36)
- ✓ Stimulates the Immune System: Triggers the immune system, helps with flushing of toxins, stimulates blood circulation and purification.
- ✓ Mood: Known to be grounding, balancing and warming, it is a good one for cleansing the air and creating a protective and warm environment.
- ✓ IBS: blend turmeric with an oil and massage on the tummy. Alternate with peppermint, or blend the two.
- ✓ Massage for fatigue or post-viral recovery: Turmeric is excellent for a gentle, soothing massage, easy on the senses. It can help recovery after a viral infection.
- ✓ Cut or wound healing: Blend 4 drops turmeric with 5 drops lavender to help heal skin and wound.
- ✓ Stimulant for the Liver: Can help with sluggish digestion, liver congestion and cleansing, but to be used in moderation and during short periods for this purpose.

WARNING: Excessive turmeric can act as a blood thinner, so avoid overuse or use sparingly (with doctor approval) if on blood-clotting meds. Avoid during pregnancy.

Dr. Schnaubelt writes that it may have the ability to interfere with cell signaling pathways, used in the treatment of squamous cell carcinoma and melanoma as well as other cancers. (34)

Valerie Wormwood, in her book The Fragrant Mind, calls the personality of turmeric a “Rootie” (like ginger and vetiver). She says that it is easy to pass the rooties by unnoticed, as they don’t have the flamboyance of a floral or the drive of other personalities. They have gracious, grounded qualities, solid and strong. (35)

Dr. Axe points to more than 7000 peer-reviewed studies on curcumin, turmeric’s active ingredient. (36)

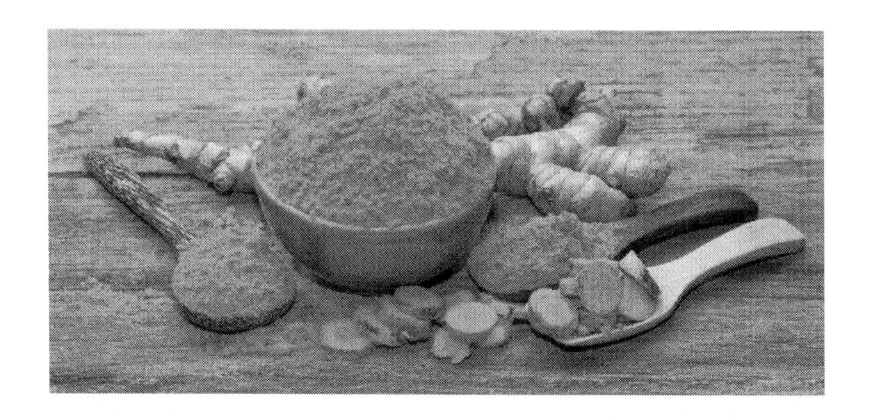

Chapter 9

SOME SIMPLE & HELPFUL BLENDING RECIPES + TYPICAL DILUTIONS

"The best and most efficient pharmacy is within your system." - Robert C. Peale

"He who has health, has hope; and he who has hope, has everything." -Thomas Carlyle

Please note, I wrote a full book of recipes and methods called USE THIS FOR THAT! YOUR EASY ESSENTIAL OIL GUIDEBOOK. This book can be helpful if you are ready to dive into the real everyday uses of your essential oils and get the most benefit from them - and it'ss far more detailed that just the few basics found in this chapter.

Similar to the philosophy of keeping it simple by listing my top essential oils, I want to provide some simple and helpful essential oil recipes for you here.

There are plenty of books, websites and aromatherapists who provide recipes for every condition known to man! We are focused here for you, and provide a jumping off spot.

First, let's address Dilutions and Dosages:

Recommendations on dilutions and dosages of essential oil (from Aromahead):

There are approximately 500–600 drops per oz of essential oil. The dilution guidelines are based on this number.

1% of 500 = 5 1% of 600 = 6.

Use the following dilutions for problems that are emotional in nature, for accessing the subtle energetic effects of the oils, for pregnant women and children, for anyone with a compromised immune system, and for using directly on the face:

1% dilution = 5–6 drops total of essential oil in 1 oz (30 ml) of carrier. If you are using three different oils, this might translate into 2 drops of each oil in the blend.

For massage oils and daily use: 2% dilution = 10–12 total drops of essential oil in 1 oz (30 ml) carrier.

For specific injury of muscle, tendon, bone: 3–10% depending on the individual, age, situation and oils being used. 3% dilution = 15–18 total drops of essential oil in 1 oz (30 ml) carrier.

For local issues such as chest congestion: 3–10% depending on the individual, age, situation and oils being used.

If the problem is **acute and severe, you can go up to 25% dilution** for very short term use, but this is rare. (These problems include severe muscle cramps, intense spasms in the moment, significant bruising, or pain.)

"Neat" (this means undiluted essential oil and no carrier oil) oils can be used for the following: Small areas, local use, acute situations, short-term use. These must be the highest quality, non-oxidized oils, and can be used in steams. (Acute situations include headache, superficial cuts, bee sting, bug bite, burn.)

1 oz (30 ml) of carrier

1% Dilution: 5–6 drops total
2% Dilution: 10–12 drops total
3% Dilution: 15–18 drops total

2 oz (60 ml) of carrier

1% Dilution: 10–12 drops total
2% Dilution: 20–24 drops total
3% Dilution: 30–36 drops total

Carrier Oils and Tools

To Blend, you need a Carrier Oil, a bowl, the sealable bottle for your finished product (amber or blue) or inhaler (we love these URL LINK) or jar you will use for your finished product – and your Essential Oils! Some use a funnel. (I haven't found the need.)

Carrier Oils – we recommend always buying a Certified Organic oil. If not, you risk using an oil with pesticides, additives, dyes and other things that will be absorbed into your body system. Keep it pure!

Our favorite oils for blending are:

- Jojoba (technically a wax ester) which is close to our skin's sebum and is a great carrier agent;

- Baobab oil, extremely hardy, long-term oil that resists rancidity and if chock full of vitamins and minerals. It is rich, a preferred massage oil and wonderful for topical use.

- Depending on the use, Coconut oil, Sesame or Sunflower can be excellent as well!

When dropping in the essential oils to the recipe, try to follow the recommended drops but don't worry if you put a few more or less in. It is hard to control, and a drop or 2 more won't make a big difference.

BASIC RECIPES

We typically recommend the following: if you are going to use a topical (a blended recipe smoothed on the body with an oil or cream, or essential oils on a compress, or "neat" for instance), always inhale it directly first. Bioavailability is better with inhalation, meaning more effective and swifter action in that route, but in many instances, topical is also useful as it works slower and lasts longer the skin. In other words, for most applications calling for a topical, it makes sense to also inhale.

INSOMNIA

1) Simply diffuse lavender at night in the bedroom. Simplicity at its best.

In addition, you could add a few lavender drops to your washing machine when you wash your sheets and pillowcases; you could put a few drops of lavender on a cotton ball or in a sachet and tuck it under the pillow.

2) Blend 10 drops lavender, 10 drops Roman chamomile, 4 drops vetiver and 4 drops clary sage in an ounce of carrier oil. Apply on neck, wrists and feet at night and inhale or diffuse. (I like to use the rollerball applicators in a glass bottle – easy when you are tired at night and effective.)

3) Buy a premade Sleep Blend. Many companies offer them (including mine). Our Zen Sublime Sleep is blended in an organic carrier oil so it can be applied to your skin as well as inhaled or diffused. Here is the blend and why I chose each EO:

- **Lavender** – well known and most used essential oil for sleep assistance. Lavender calms, soothes and nurtures. It helps to balance the spirit, and reduces any existing anxiety. It also helps reduce pains which may hinder sleep.

- **Rose Geranium** – fosters a sense of security and protects from disturbing energy or thoughts.
- **Orange** – unblocks energy; found in clinical tests to be a sedative that calms, pushes down pessimism and is a tonic for mind and body.
- **Neroli** – relaxes nerves, soothes the heart and psyche, and helps relieve pain.
- **Cedarwood** – is very grounding, a tonic for the nervous system and is of course anti-inflammatory.
- **Clary Sage** – well-known to reduce anxiety and stress, which may be the cause of sleeplessness. It works synergistically with lavender for sedation and calming effect.

SORE THROAT

1) Do a steam inhalation of 2 drops Chamomile, 3 drops Lavender and 1 drop Thyme.

2) For simplicity, do a steam inhalation of just 2 drops Clove.

After a steam inhalation, massage the blend of 2 drops Lemon, 1 drop Thyme and 4 drops Chamomile in a tablespoon of a carrier oil onto your throat and neck (including behind your ears.)

3) (*From Aromahead*) Put one drop of Tea Tree in a glass of warm water, mix it, and then gargle. Don't

worry if you swallow a little, but try to spit out most of it. Gargle like this several times a day. You can also put one drop of Sandalwood in a bit of jojoba and rub it on the front and back of your neck.

4) Make this blend to inhale or diffuse every 3 hours. 12 drops lavender, 6 drops black pepper and 3 drops myrrh.

5) Buy a premade blend. There are many available!

6) I personally find that if a sore throat is making it's appearance and hasn't really taken hold, I inhale Eucalyptus every hour (and sometimes I will also inhale myrrh and/or clove) and it goes away.

TONSILLITIS

1) Blend in 2 teaspoons of a carrier oil 6 drops Rose Geranium, 4 drops Myrrh and 2 drops Orange or Sweet Orange. Massage on the throat and neck, and inhale.

2) Put 1 drop of Tea Tree in 1 tsp of honey plus 1 cup of warm water, mix well then gargle (do not swallow.)

COUGH

1) Blend 2 drops Eucalyptus, 2 drops lemon and 1 drop Tea Tree in 2 teaspoons honey. Dilute in a cup of warm water and gargle.

2a) For a spasmodic cough: blend 2 drops Cypress and 1 drop Frankincense on a cotton ball or tissue, inhale deeply.

2b) For a spasmodic cough (*from Aromahead)*: blend 5 drops Black Pepper, 5 drops Frankincense and 5 drops Black Spruce in a personal handheld inhaler. Use as needed.

3) Dry cough: Mix Eucalyptus 3 drops, and Thyme 2 drops in 1 teaspoon of a carrier, massage on chest and throat.

4) Blend Eucalyptus, Cedarwood, Pine and Myrrh in 1/6 ounce bottle. Inhale, use in a diffuser or tent steam; or mix with a carrier oil 1 ounce and massage on the throat.

TOOTH ACHE

1) Dot Clove onto a Q-tip and touch the affected area. It will help reduce pain and inflammation.

CONGESTION

1) Do a Eucalyptus steam. Add 10 drops of Eucalyptus and 10 drops of Siberian Fir Needle with 8 drops of Tea Tree and 2 drops Myrrh to boiling water. Make a steam tent with a towel and inhale with eyes closed.

2) Put 2-4 drops of Eucalyptus in the corner of your shower in the morning, and let the steam rise and help you. Make sure to put the drops where you won't stand or step to avoid slipping.

3) Blend Eucalyptus, Myrrh, Peppermint and Lemon or diffuse any one of these (your choice) to help break

up congestion and breathe better. They will also clarify the air.

4) Buy a premade blend that can be massaged on your chest and throat as well as inhaled. Ours is blended in organic jojoba and sunflower and includes:

- **Eucalyptus** - well-known and wide ranging benefits, including sinus and respiratory applications, increases blood flow and helps with mental exhaustion. It is known to be anti-inflammatory, antispasmodic and very importantly, a decongestant.
- **Rosemary** - In addition decreasing the levels of cortisol (a stress hormone which can kick in when you are sick which hurts the immune system), Rosemary oil has properties believed to be helpful in relieving respiratory issues and reducing pain.
- **Juniper Berry** - among its many qualities, Juniper Berry is a detoxifer or purifer of blood, helping to remove toxins.
- **Lime** - Limes, like lemons, are full of antioxidants, bactericides and other beneficial nutrients. It helps to fight and protect against viral infections which may cause the common cold. Additionally, lime is an antiseptic, meaning it can cure infections and protect against their development.

HEADACHE

There are different types of headaches, from a sinus headache, migraine to a tension headache. Here are a few suggestions:

1) For many types of headaches, use a cool compress or washcloth. Swish the cloth in cool water with 2 drops lavender and 1 drop peppermint, or 2 drops lavender and 1 drop Rose Geranium (inhale to see what you react to better). Put the cold compress on your forehead and relax in a darkened room.

2) General headache for no reason: 3 drops Lavender and 1 drop peppermint, use neat or blend in 1 tsp of a carrier. Apply and massage around the temples, back of neck and around the hairline (be sure to patch test first any EO used neat.)

3) Nervous headache: 3 drops lavender and 2 drops chamomile or an alternative is 1 drop Rose Geranium, 2 drops lemon and 3 drops lavender in 1 tsp of a carrier. Massage in and relax.

4) Sinus headache: steam inhale 3 drops rosemary, 1 drop thyme and 1 drop peppermint or eucalyptus.

5) Acute sinusitis: Combine 4 drops eucalyptus, lavender, peppermint, pine and tea tree in a bowl, drop in a wick for an inhaler or cotton balls, then place inside the personal inhaler and use 5 times a day.

Do the same recipe but only 1 drop of each in hot water and do a steam inhalation.

In a pinch, inhale eucalyptus directly from the bottle frequently.

6) Tension headache: Blend into 1 ounce of cream 3 drops lavender, 4 drops Frankincense, 1 drop Rosemary and 1 drop Helichrysum. Run on the back of your neck and temples when tension begins.

7) General headache: Put 4 drops of lemon in 1 tsp of carrier, and drop in a bath and relax in the tub.

8) Buy a premade blend, made by many companies.

ANXIETY ATTACK

1) Blend 10 drops each of Lavender, Geranium and Rosemary and diffuse or inhale.

2) Blend Neroli 7 drops, Lavender 3 drops and Lemon 20 drops; diffuse.

3) For guilt & depression that spurs anxiety: 15 drops Rose Geranium, 10 drops Bergamot, Lavender 5 drops, Turmeric 5 drops; diffuse.

4) Inhale or diffuse Rosemary or Lavender alone.

PLAIN OLD STRESS

1) Blend 3 drops Lavender, 3 drops Bergamot, 1 drop Rose Geranium and 1 drop Frankincense in a diffuser or personal inhaler.

2) Blend 3 drops of Clary Sage, 1 drop of Lemon and 1 drop Lavender in your diffuser or personal inhaler.

3) Massage Blend. Blend into 1 ounce of a carrier oil 5 drops Cedarwood, 5 drops Bergamot, 2 drops Jasmine or Ylang Ylang and 1 drop Neroli.

4) Buy a premade blend. We love ours – Zen De-Stress is blended in organic jojoba and sunflower oil, and includes:

- **Lavender** – lavender essential oil has the ability to eliminate nervous tension, relieve and calm. The refreshing aroma also helps with nervous exhaustion and helps lower blood pressure.
- **Clary Sage** – is an anti-depressant among its many powers. It helps fight depression and relieves anxiety while helping to boost joy.
- **Neroli** – is also an anti-depressant along with holding sedative powers. It helps drive away sadness and lifts the mood (which is why this oil is extensively used in Aromatherapy techniques.)
- **Roman Chamomile** – is excellent for combating stress, and helps those who are depressed, lonely or fearful. It helps calm, and is also good for times of anger or irritability.

TUMMY RUB FOR CONSTIPATION *(from Aromahead)*

1) Blend into 1 ounce of cream 7 drops Sweet Marjoram, 3 drops Bergamot, 3 drops Orange, 2 drops Neroli, 1 drop Roman Chamomile and 5 drops Spikenard. Massage on tummy several times daily.

TUMMY RUB FOR IBS OR CRAMPS *(from Aromahead)*

1) Blend into 2 ounces of a cream 5 drops of Orange, 5 drops Roman Chamomile, 5 drops Sandalwood and 4 drops Bergamot. Massage on belly and lower back every few hours.

2) Blend 6 drops Turmeric into a carrier oil. (Add 2 drops Bergamot if desired) Massage on tummy.

3) Blend 2-3 drops Clove and 4 drops Roman Chamomille into a carrier oil and massage onto your tummy. Can also help relieve gas

BLISS AND RELAXATION

1) For an uplifting yet blissful feeling, blend into 1 ounce of cream or oil 2 drops Rose Geranium, 2 drops Bergamot, 1 drop Orange.

3) Buy a premade blend. Our Zen Air Bliss contains: Ylang Ylang, Sweet Orange, Bergamot, Magnolia and Neroli.

MUSCLE PAIN AND STIFFNESS

1) Blend into 1 ounce of a carrier like jojoba or baobab: 4 drops Eucalyptus, 4 drops Black Pepper, 4 drops Lavender and 2 drops Rosemary. Rub on the affected area as needed (every 2 hours when there is acute pain.)

2) You can put the same recipe on a compress without the carrier (cool or warm). Drop the essential

oils into a bowl of water (heated or cooled), swish your cloth in it, wring out and apply. For extra power, put your carrier solution on the skin; then apply the compress.

SWOLLEN MUSCLES AND JOINTS

1) Blend into 1 ounce of a carrier oil 8 drops Roman Chamomile, 3 drops Lavender, 4 drops Frankincense, 3 drops Helichrysum.

2) Simplicity for arthritis or rheumatoid arthritis: use Frankincense or Turmeric, or blend both in an oil or cream; twice daily, massage into the affected joints. Diffuse Frankincense or Turmeric when desired.

CUTS

1) Put 1-2 drops of Lavender neat on the cut, or

2) Put 1-2 drops of Helichrysum neat on the cut, or

3) Put 1-2 drops of Rose Geranium on the cut.

Each will serve as an antibacterial and healing agent. Rose Geranium has a clotting action and helps stop the bleeding. (I keep these 3 in the kitchen for handy use.) Turmeric does the same thing, and is good as a followup for healing in a gel or cream.

LEG CRAMPS

1) Blend 2 drops Peppermint, 4 drops Cypress, 2 drops Ginger, and 2 drops Sweet Marjoram with 4 teaspoons carrier oil of your choice and massage in.

2) Blend into 15 ml of Coconut oil or other carrier oil 5 drops Rosemary oil, 3 drops Lavender oil, 2 drops Turmeric and 6 drops Marjoram oil. Massage in circular motions.

3) In a pinch, simply blend Peppermint in jojoba oil and massage in.

Check if your calcium, magnesium and potassium levels are off or not in balance. This could cause cramps, among other things.

COLD SORES

1) (*courtesy Aromahead.*) Blend 30 drops Sandalwood and 3 drops Eucalyptus radiate into 1 ounce of aloe vera gel. Dab it on the cold sore or area where it is developing ever hour.

ACNE

Tea Tree and Juniper Berry are two essential oils that have been studied and tested with acne. Tea Tree is effective on acne and oily skin, and juniper berry is a good antibacterial for acne.

1) Tea Tree could be used "neat" but do the patch test first. Simply drop 2-3 drops of Tea Tree onto the acne or pimple twice daily. Otherwise, blend into jojoba which works with well with the skin.

2) Blend Tea Tree and Juniper into an aloe gel or jojoba oil, and use as a serum to tamp down oil and breakouts.

PESTS (Mice, rats, cockroaches)

These pests hate or fear Peppermint. Put 4-5 drops of Peppermint on a tea bag and place at the back of kitchen cabinets or where there may be holes in the wall or cabinets (points of entry) as a deterrent. Likewise, Clove is helpful against spiders and bugs. Make sure your dog or cat can't get at the tea bag!

REFRESHING YOUR HOME

We have mentioned some uses throughout the book. Here are just a few of them:

Put 2 drops of Lavender in your washing machine or a 1 drop on the dryer cloth when doing bed linens – or any laundry!

Put 1 drop of Lavender in your dishwasher to help disinfect and freshen.

Use your favorite essential oil (Lemon, Lime or Bergamot work well) to wipe down surfaces. Put drops into spray bottle with water or white vinegar.

Use Tea Tree on a paper towel to wipe around areas that get fungi or mold (inside hidden areas of washer, drains, bathroom corners.

Diffuse your favorite essential oils in various rooms for various situation, such as: energetic children at night – diffuse lavender an hour before bedtime (and in the bedroom if desired). Sick ones at home – diffuse clove or eucalyptus or lemon. Want a tranquil environment – diffuse frankincense. A joyful one – do a blend like Zen Bliss, or diffuse sweet orange, ylang ylang, frankincense or bergamot. Grieving – diffuse Rose Geranium. Diffuse your favorite essential oil.

There are hundreds more recipes and uses for essential oils, and I hope this has given you a jumping off point!

Chapter 10

CARING FOR YOUR ESSENTIAL OILS

Having good health is very different from only being not sick.

~ Seneca The Younger, 50 AD

Essential oils will have an average life of about 18 - 24 months under the following conditions (though they could go longer if well cared for as below). Top tips:

- ✓ They are in a darker bottle, typically amber or blue, to protect from light
- ✓ They are kept in an airtight bottle (meaning the top isn't loose or you forgot to close the lid tightly – oxygen is not a friend of these volatile essential oils and is its WORST enemy!)
- ✓ They are typically kept in a cooler, darker space – certainly avoid exposing them direct sunlight or heat.
- ✓ Robert Tisserand and other experts recommend keeping your essential oils in a

fridge for the longest life possible. If you keep them next to food, it's best to put the oils in a zip lock bag or a container, as the scents could pass to food. If you have a separate half-fridge in your house, basement or garage, it could serve you well!

TO SUMMARIZE

Purchase essential oils only if they come in dark bottles, typically blue or brown glass.

If you are making some blends yourself, put the new blends into blue or amber glass bottles. Plastic will be "melted" by essential oils and it will ruin your blend. Don't use plastic.

Light and heat reduce the effectiveness of essential oils and shorten its life. When you use an oil, open it – use it – seal it tight. Don't leave a bottle open as you mix and blend, or set up the diffuser, or answer the phone.

Oxygen inside a bottle can eventually cause color deterioration and rancid odor.

Ideal temperature? 40 to 60 degrees Fahrenheit (5 to 20 degrees Celsius) but if you are using an essential oil frequently, and keep it in a room that is warmer, OK. Just keep it out of direct light. I keep my extras in a fridge (I have one of the little half-size fridges dedicated to essential oils and some skincare) but the ones I am currently diffusing on a shelf in the office; several in the bathroom; and several in the kitchen for cuts. I keep a lavender bottle in the laundry room as well.

I personally like to buy essential oils whereby a GC/MS test is available, and I offer the same test to any client who buys our products. The purpose is to see the makeup and constituents, but also to verify against dilution or alteration. As an everyday buyer, you may not do this, but then stick with companies that you trust and get on with it!

I hope you are enjoying your discovery of essential oils, whether for healing, beauty, cleaning, protection, or helping solve everyday issues. And I hope this book will help you and your loved ones gain more understanding and become more empowered!

REFERENCES

Safety First

1) Robert Tisserand and Rodney Young, PhD. Essential Oil Safety: A Guide for Healthcare Professionals. 2nd edition. Churchill Livingstone Publishers

Chapter 1 What are These Things called Essential Oils, and Why Do They Have Super Powers?

1) http://ensia.com/features/banned-in-europe-safe-in-the-u-s/

2) http://www.newsmax.com/Health/Health-News/obesity-weight-loss-DrAlan-Hirsch-SENSA/2013/03/31/id/497088/

3) NAHA seminar on Pharmacology Basics, February 2016

4) Serafino, A., Vallebona et al. Stimulatory effect of Eucalyptus essential oil on innate cell-mediated immune response. 2008. BMC Immunology.

5a) Ledoux, JE. Rationalizing Thoughtless Emotions, Insight, Sept. 1989

5b) Hirsch, AR, Inhalation of Odorants for Weight Reduction, Int J Obes, 1994, page 306

6) Godfrey, Heather. BSc (Joint Hons) PGCE, MIFA. "THE ROLE OF ESSENTIAL OILS IN THE TREATMENT AND MANAGEMENT OF ATTENTION DEFICIT HYPERACTIVE

DISORDER (ADHD)". Originally published in The International Journal of Aromatherapy (2001): Harcourt Publishers Ltd: vol 11 no. 4. Reviewed by the author January 2009

7) Nasel, 1992

8) Tisserand & Balacs, 1995.

9) NAHA seminar on Pharmacology Basics, February 2016

10) Robert Tisserand and Rodney Young, PhD. Essential Oil Safety: A Guide for Healthcare Professionals. 2nd edition. Churchill Livingstone Publishers

11) http://articles.mercola.com/sites/articles/archive/2016/02/18/psychological-states-influence-immune-function.aspx

12) Medical News Today. http://www.medicalnewstoday.com/articles/305921.php?page=2

13) Dr. Joie Power. NAHA talk.

Chapter 2 Fascinating History of Aromatic Plants & Essential Oils

1) Rolf Deininger, "The Magic World of Essential Oils and Scents, Their Influence on the Psyche. Wholistic Aromatherapy, A Scientific Conference on Therapeutic Uses of Essential Oils. 1995.

2) Lawless J., Aromatherapy and the Mind. 1994.

3) p 86, Gattefossé's Aromatherapy, 1937.)

4) http://www.woundsresearch.com/article/8088

5) Ayurveda, 2015.

6) Gloria McBreen

7) http://www.suzannebovenizer.com/aromatherapy-essential-oils/history

8) http://www.bbc.com/news/uk-england-nottinghamshire-32117815

9) http://www.encyclopedia.com/topic/Philippus_Aureolus_Paracelsus.aspx

10) http://tisserandinstitute.org/infographic-essential-oils-as-antimicrobials/

11) (Nicholas Culpeper, The English Physician, 1653. online through Yale Medical Library: http://www.med.yale.edu/library/historical/culpeper/culpeper.htm)

12) http://www.jonnsaromatherapy.com/history2.html

13) Gattefosse book or else Tisserand's book.

14) Bio/Tech News, 2014.

15) Steinman & Epstein, 1995

16) Schnaubelt, Dr. Kurt. The Healing Intelligence of Essential Oils. 2011.

17) IBID page 26

18) IBID

Chapter 3 The Wow Factor: Clinical Research and Studies of Essential

1) http://tisserandinstitute.org/infographic-essential-oils-as-antimicrobials/

2) Schnaubelt, Dr. Kurt. The Healing Intelligence of Essential Oils: The Science of Advanced Aromatherapy. Healing Arts Press. 2011. pg 13.

3) Valerie Ann Worwood. The Fragrant Mind. New World Library. page 6.

4) IAMA Life. http://www.iamalife.org/tag/clinical-research/

5 Valnet, J. (1980). The Practice of Aromatherapy. Healing Arts, Rochester, VT

6) Balz, Rodolphe. (1999). The Healing Power of Essential Oils: Fragrance Secrets for Everyday Use. p 56.

7) http://www.breathoflifeonline.com/essential-oils-to-the-rescue/

8) ibid

9) Schnaubelt, Dr. Kurt. The Healing Intelligence of Essential Oils.

10) http://ireport.cnn.com/docs/DOC-1134608

11) http://www.ncbi.nlm.nih.gov/pubmed/12143909

12) http://ireport.cnn.com/docs/DOC-1134608

13) http://drericz.com/frankincense-oil-kills-cancer-and-boosts-immunity/

14) http://www.greenmedinfo.com/blog/frankincense-superior-chemotherapy-killing-late-stage-ovarian-cancer-cells

Chapter 4 The Crisis of "Super Bugs", Antibiotics and Essential Oils

1) http://www.usatoday.com/story/news/nation/2013/03/05/superbugs-infections-hospitals/1965133/

2) http://www.ncbi.nlm.nih.gov/pmc/articles/PMC3109405/

3) http://www.theatlantic.com/health/archive/2015/01/the-new-antibiotics-might-be-essential-oils/384247/

4) http://www.bbc.com/news/health-28098838

5)
http://www.usatoday.com/story/news/nation/2013/03/05/superbugs-infections-hospitals/1965133/

6) ibid

7A)
http://www.theatlantic.com/health/archive/2015/01/the-new-antibiotics-might-be-essential-oils/384247/

7B) Neu, Dr. Harold. Science Magazine. "The crisis in antibiotic resistance." 1992.

7C) Schmidt, Michael A. "Antibiotics: The Promise and the Peril", a paper presented at the 1st Wholistic Aromatherapy Conference November 1995. Kurt Schnaubelt, Editor.

8) http://www.medicinehunter.com/dr-jim-duke/

9A)
https://www.researchgate.net/publication/11968992_Percutaneous_treatment_of_chronic_MRSA_osteomyelitis_with_a_novel_plant-derived_antiseptic

9B) Harrison, Jimm. "Intravenous Administration of Essential Oils", a paper presented for Unlimited Possibilities: Proceedings of the 8th International Aromatherapy Conference. Nov 2015. Schnaubelt, Dr. Kurt (Editor).

10) Anderson JN, Fennessy PA: Can tea tree (Melaleuca alternifolia) oil prevent MRSA? Medical Journal of Australia 2000, 173:489

11) http://www.drweil.com/drw/u/WBL02195/Herbal-Oils-Thwart-Germs.html

12) https://www.sciencedaily.com/releases/2010/03/100330210942.htm

13) Edwards-Jones, V., Buck, R., Shawcross S.G., Dawson, M.M. and Dunn, K. (2004) The effect of essential oils on methicillin-resistant Staphylococcus aureus using a dressing model. Burns 30, 8, 772-777.

14) http://tisserandinstitute.org/resistance-is-futile/

15) http://tisserandinstitute.org/resistance-is-futile/

16) http://www.readcube.com/articles/10.4172%2F2329-8731.1000105

17) http://phys.org/news/2010-03-essential-oils-superbugs.html

18) Lancet. Allen, P. 2001, 358

19) http://www.ncbi.nlm.nih.gov/pubmed/22257599

20) http://www.ncbi.nlm.nih.gov/pubmed/23445470

21) "Essential Oils, A New Horizon in Combating Bacterial Antibiotic Resistance." http://www.ncbi.nlm.nih.gov/pmc/articles/PMC3950955/

22) http://tisserandinstitute.org/infographic-essential-oils-as-antimicrobials/

23) Tori Rodriguez, Jan 16, 2015. "Essential Oils Might Be the New Antibiotics." The Atlantic. http://www.theatlantic.com/health/archive/2015/01/the-new-antibiotics-might-be-essential-oils/384247/

24) http://www.ncbi.nlm.nih.gov/pmc/articles/PMC3109405/

25) http://www.ncbi.nlm.nih.gov/pubmed/17127526

26) http://ps.oxfordjournals.org/content/86/11/2466.full

27) http://articles.mercola.com/sites/articles/archive/2016/03/19/antibiotic-use-agriculture.aspx?e_cid=20160319Z1_DNL_art_1&utm_source=dnl&utm_medium=email&utm_content=art1&utm_campaign=20160319Z1&et_cid=DM100455&et_rid=1408602215

28) Tori Rodriguez, Jan 16, 2015. "Essential Oils Might Be the New Antibiotics." The Atlantic. http://www.theatlantic.com/health/archive/2015/01/the-new-antibiotics-might-be-essential-oils/384247/

29) Tori Rodriguez, Jan 16, 2015. "Essential Oils Might Be the New Antibiotics." The Atlantic. http://www.theatlantic.com/health/archive/2015/01/the-new-antibiotics-might-be-essential-oils/384247/

30) Cari Romm. Oct 3, 2014 The FDA Says Farmers Are Giving Animals Too Many Antibiotics. http://www.theatlantic.com/health/archive/2014/10/american-meat-has-more-antibiotics-than-ever/381100/

31) http://www.theatlantic.com/health/archive/2015/01/the-new-antibiotics-might-be-essential-oils/384247/

32) "Essential oils key to Cargill's comprehensive approach to reducing antibiotics in poultry". January 27, 2016. http://www.cargill.com/news/releases/2016/NA31925706.jsp

33) http://www.ncbi.nlm.nih.gov/pmc/articles/PMC3109405/

Chapter 5 Different Approaches to Essential Oils Around the World

1) Schnaubelt, Dr. Kurt. The Healing Intelligence of Essential Oils. Healing Arts Press, Rochester VT. 2011. pg 111

2) ibid. pg 11-12

3) Schnaubelt, Dr. Kurt. Medical Aromatherapy, Healing with Essential Oils. Frog, Ltd. Berkeley. page 60.

4)
http://www.atlanticinstitute.com/blog/2014/7/14/schools-myth-draft

5) Schnaubelt, Dr. Kurt. The Healing Intelligence of Essential Oils. Healing Arts Press, Rochester VT. 2011. pg 93

6) http://patient.info/doctor/complementary-and-alternative-medicine

7) http://www.thelancet.com/

8) http://www.huffingtonpost.com/dana-ullman/homeopathic-medicine-_b_1258607.html

9) http://www.huffingtonpost.com/dana-ullman/abraham-lincoln-homeopathy_b_2177808.html

Chapter 6 Mind – Body – Spirit and Aromatherapy

1) Dr. Mark Hyman. Functional Wellness, Part 5: the Mind-Body Connection.
https://experiencelife.com/article/functional-wellness-part-5-the-body-mind-connection/

2)
http://articles.mercola.com/sites/articles/archive/2016/02/18/psychological-states-influence-immune-function.aspx

3)
http://articles.mercola.com/sites/articles/archive/2012/04/11/epigenetic-vs-determinism.aspx

4) http://www.drweil.com/drw/u/id/ART02741

5) Patricia Davis. Aromatherapy A-Z. 1988. pg 173

6) Valerie Ann Worwood. The Fragrant Mind. pg 39.

7) ibid

8) Science March 21 2014

9) American Spa, Sept 2015. Nicole Altavilla.

10) http://articles.mercola.com/sites/articles/archive/2014/09/04/essential-oils-aromatherapy.aspx#_edn18

11) http://articles.mercola.com/sites/articles/archive/2012/04/11/epigenetic-vs-determinism.aspx

12) http://www.ameo.com/media-center/zija-news/20150909/am%C3%A9o-research-development-series-gene-expression

13) Dr. Scott Johnson and Dr. Joshua Plant. Synergy, It's an Essential Oil Thing: Revealing the Science of Essential Oil Synergy with Cells, Genes and Human Health. Oct 2015.

14) ibid

15) Valerie Ann Worwood. The Fragrant Mind. pg 31

16) Dr. David Stewart. Quantum Physics, Essential Oils and the Mind-Body Connection: How Essential Oils Really Work. 2008 by Soundconcepts.

Chapter 7 The Magic of Extraction... and a Little Science (the Main Components in Oils Which Give Them Powers)

1) Quantum Physics, Essential Oils and the Mind-Body Connection. Dr. David Stewart, Ph.D. Brochure published by Soundconcepts. 2008.

Chapter 8 My Top 15 Essential Oils, Benefits and Properties

1) Greenway, F.L., Frome, B.M., Engels, T.M. and McLellan, A. (2003) Temporary relief of postherpetic neuralgia pain with topical geranium oil. American Journal of Medicine 115, 7, 586-587.

2) Edwards-Jones, V., Buck, R., Shawcross S.G., Dawson, M.M. and Dunn, K. (2004) The effect of essential oils on methicillin-resistant Staphylococcus aureus using a dressing model. Burns 30, 8, 772-777.

3) Buchbauer, G. (1993) Biological Effects and Modes of Action of Essential Oils. International Journal of Aromatherapy 5, 1, 11-14.

4) Fu, Y.-J., Zu, Y.-G., Chen, L.-Y., Shi, X.-G., Wang, Z., Sun, S. and Efferth, T. (2007) Antimicrobial activity of clove and rosemary essential oils alone and in combination. Phytotherapy Research 21, 989-994.

5) Tragoolpua, Y. and Jaatisatienr, A. (2007) Anti-herpes simplex virus activities of Eugenia caryophyllus (Spreng.) Bullock & S. G. Harrison and essential oil, eugenol. Phytotherapy Research 21, 12, 1153-1158.

6) Toni VanGils – Director Aromatherapy Institute, quotes from an article in the AEI newsletter circulated on Sheri Nakken's vaccine information list.

(7) Tisserand and Young 2014 + Bodake, H., Panicker, K., Kailaje, V. and Rao, V. (2002) Chemopreventative effect of orange oil on the development of hepatic preneoplastic lesions induced by N-nitrosodiethylamine in rats: an ultrastructural study. Indian Journal of Experimental Biology 40, 245-251 (2002) + Ozbek, H., Ugras, S., Dulger, H., Bayram, I., Tuncer, I., Oztürk, G. and Oztürk, A. (2003) Hepatoprotective effect of Foeniculum vulgare essential oil. Fitoterapia 74, 3, 317-319. Notes that d-limonene had hepatoprotective action.

8) Hongratanaworakit,T. (2009) Simultaneous aromatherapy massage with rosemary oil on humans. Scientica Pharmaceutica 77, 375-387.

9) Moss, M. and Oliver, L. (2012) Plasma 1,8-cineole correlates with cognitive performance following exposure to rosemary essential oil aroma. Therapeutic Advances in Psychopharmacology 2, 3, 103-113.

10) Fu, Y.-J., Zu, Y.-G., Chen, L.-Y., Shi, X.-G., Wang, Z., Sun, S. and Efferth, T. (2007) Antimicrobial activity of clove and

rosemary essential oils alone and in combination. Phytotherapy Research 21, 989-994.

11) Sinha, P., Srivastava, Mishra, N. and Yadav, N.P. (2014) New perspectives on antiacne plant drugs: contribution to modern therapeutics. BioMed Research International. Article ID 301304. Available at http://dx.doi.org/10.1155/2014/301304

12) Edwards-Jones, V., Buck, R., Shawcross S.G., Dawson, M.M. and Dunn, K. (2004) The effect of essential oils on methicillin-resistant Staphylococcus aureus using a dressing model. Burns 30, 8, 772-777.

13) Edris, A.E. (2007) Pharmaceutical and therapeutic potentials of essential oils and their individual volatile constituents: a review. Phytotherapy Research 21, 308-323.

14) Garozzo, A., Timpanaro, R., Bisignano, B., Furneri, P.M., Bisignano, G. and Castro, A. (2009) In vitro antiviral activity of Melaleuca alternifolia essential oil. Letters in Applied Microbiology 49, 6, 806-808.

15 Hongratanaworakit, T. and Buchbauer, G. (2004) Evaluation of the harmonizing effect of ylang ylang on humans after inhalation. Planta Medica 70, 7, 632-636. + Hongratanaworakit, T. and Buchbauer, G. (2006) Relaxing effect of ylang ylang on humans after transdermal absorption. Phytotherapy Research 20, 9, 758-763.

16) Hwang, J.H. (2006) The effects of the inhalation method using essential oils on blood pressure and stress responses of clients with essential hypertension. Taehan Kanhoe Hakhoe Chi 36, 7, 1123-1134. Article in Korean. Available at
http://www.ncbi.nim.nih.gov/pubmed/17211115

17) Weiss, E.A. (1997) Essential Oil Crops. Wallingford: CAB International.

18) Su, S., Wang, T., Duan, J.A., Zhou, W., Hua, Y.Q., Tang, Y.P., Yu, L. and Qian, D.W. (2011) Anti-inflammatory and analgesic activity of different extracts of Commiphora myrrha. Journal of Ethnopharmacology 134, 251-258.

19) Shen, T., Li, G.H., Wang, X.N. and Lou, H.X. (2012) The genus Commiphora: a review of its traditional uses, phytochemistry and pharmacology. Journal of Ethnopharmacology 142, 2, 319-330.

20) Tonkal, A.M. and Morsy, T.A. (2008) An update review on Commiphora molmol and related species. Journal of the Egyptian Society of Parasitology 38, 3, 763-796.

21) Voinchet, V. and Giraud-Robert, A.-M. (2007) Utilisation de l'huile essentielle d'hélichryse italienne et de l'huile végétale de rose musquée après intervention de chirurgie plastique réparatrice et esthétique. Phytothérapie 2, 67-72.

22) Lorenzi, V., Muselli, A., Bernardini, A.F., Berti, L., Pagès, J.-M., Amaral, L. and Bola, J.-M. (2009) Geraniol restores

antibiotic activities against multidrug-resistant isolates from Gram-negative species. Antimicrobial Agents and Chemotherapy 53, 5, 2209-2211.

23) Jirovetz, L., Eller, G., Buchbauer, G., Schmidt, E., Denkova, Z., Stoyanova, A.S., Nikolova, R., Geissler, M. (2006) Chemical composition, antimicrobial activities, and odor descriptions of some essential oils with characteristic floral-rosy scent and of their principal aroma compounds. Recent Developments in Agronomy & Horticulture 2, 1-12.

24) Nostro A, Bisignano G, Angela Cannatelli M, Crisafi G, Paola Germanò M, Alonzo V. Effects of Helichrysum italicum extract on growth and enzymatic activity of Staphylococcus aureus. 2001. http://www.ncbi.nlm.nih.gov/pubmed/11397624

25) http://www.ncbi.nlm.nih.gov/pubmed/18997985

26) http://draxe.com/helichrysum-essential-oil/

27) https://en.wikipedia.org/wiki/Bergamot_essential_oil

28) Bagetta G, Morrone LA, Rombolà L, Amatea, D, Russo R, Berliocchi L, Sakurada S, Sakurada T, Rotiroti D, Corasaniti MT (2010) Neuropharmacology of the essential oil of bergamot. Fitoterapia 81: 453-461

29) Sanguinetti M, Posteraro B, Romano L, Battaglia T, Lopizzo T, De Carolis E, Fadda G (2007). In vitro activity of Citrus bergamia (bergamot) oil against clinical isolates of

dermatophytes. Journal of Antimicrobial Chemotherapy 59 (2): 305-308

30) Romano L, Battaglia F, Masucci L, Sanguinetti M, Posteraro B, Plotti G, Zanetti S, Fadda G (2005) In vitro activity of bergamot natural essence and furocoumarins-free and distilled extracts, and their associations with boric acid, against clinical yeast isolates. Journal of Antimicrobial Chemotherapy 55 (1): 110-114

31) http://articles.mercola.com/herbal-oils/bergamot-oil.aspx

32) Hwang JH (2006) The effects of the inhalation method using essential oils on blood pressure and stress responses of clients with essential hypertension. Taehan Kanhoe Hakhoe Chi 36 (7): 1123-1134. (Article in Korean) Available at http://www.ncbi.nim.nih.gov/pubmed/17211115

33) Chang SY (2008) Effects of aroma hand massage on pain, state anxiety and depression in hospice patients with terminal cancer. Taehan Kanho Hakhoe Chi 38: 493-502 (Article in Korean). Cited by Dobetsberger C, Buchbauer G (2011) Actions of essential oils on the central nervous system: an updated review. Flavour and Fragrance Journal 26 (5): 300

34) Schnaubelt, Dr. Kurt. The Healing Intelligence of Essential Oils. Healing Arts Press. 2011. pg 162.

35) Wormwood, Valerie. The Fragrant Mind: Aromatherapy for Personality, Mind, Mood and Emotion. New World Press. 1966.

36) http://www.ncbi.nlm.nih.gov/pubmed/24513290
http://www.ncbi.nlm.nih.gov/pubmed/25159739
http://www.ncbi.nlm.nih.gov/pubmed/25173461

BIBLIOGRAPHY

Balz, Rodolphe. The Healing Power of Essential Oils. Lotus Light. 1996.

Butje, Andrea. Essential Living: Aromatherapy Recipes for Health & Home. 2nd edition. 2015.

Dodt, Colleen. The Essential Oils Book. Storey Communications, 1996.

Gattefossé, Rene-Maurice. Aromatherapy. Translated by Robert B. Tisserand. Saffron Walden, 1993.

Guenther, Ernest. The Essential Oils – Vol 1: History – Origin in Plants – Production – Analysis. D. Van Nostrand Company, 1948.

Harding, Jennie. The Essential Oils Handbook. Watkins Publishing London. 2008.

Johnson, Dr. Scott A. Evidence-Based Essential Oil Therapy. Scott A. Johnson Professional Writing Services, LLC , 2015

Johnson, Dr. Scott A. Surviving When Modern Medicine Fails. Scott A. Johnson Professional Writing Services, LLC. 2014.

Johnson, Dr. Scott A. and Plant, Dr. Joshua. Synergy, It's an Essential Oil Thing: Revealing the Science of Essential Oil Synergy with Cells, Genes and Human Health. 2015.

Lawless, Julia. The Illustrated Encyclopedia of Essential Oils. Thorsons, 1995.

Schnaubelt, Dr. Kurt. Advanced Aromatherapy. Healing Arts Press, 1998.

Schnaubelt, Dr. Kurt. The Healing Intelligence of Essential Oils. Healing Arts Press, 2011.

Schnaubelt, Dr. Kurt. Medical Aromatherapy. Frog, Ltd. 1999.

Schnaubelt, Dr. Kurt (Editor). Unlimited Possibilities: Proceedings of the 8th International Aromatherapy Conference. Nov 2015.

Stewart, Dr. David. Healing Oils of the Bible. Care Press. 2014.

Stewart, Dr. David. Quantum Physics, Essential Oils and the Mind-Body Connection (brochure). Sound Concepts, 2008.

Tisserand, Robert B. The Art of Aromatherapy. Healing Arts Press. 1977

Tisserand, Robert B. and Young, Rodney. Essential Oil Safety: A Guide for Healthcare Professionals. 2nd edition. Churchill Livingstone.

Wildwood, Chrissie. The Encyclopedia of Aromatherapy. Healing Arts Press, 2000.

Worwood, Valerie Ann. The Complete Book of Essential Oils & Aromatherapy. New World Library. 1991.

Worwood, Valerie Ann. The Fragrant Mind: Aromatherapy for Personality, Mind, Mood and Emotion. New World Library. 1996.

ABOUT THE AUTHOR

Kathy Heshelow is a busy author who also founded Sublime Naturals and Sublime Beauty – both French-inspired companies! She is working on 3 more books, two in the essential oil domain and one about aging well with French secrets and American energy.

She lived in Paris, France for 16 years, and now resides in Florida with her husband and pup.

All books are found here, including:

"Use This For That! Your Easy Essential Oil Guidebook"

"Break Sugar Cravings or Addiction, Feel Full, Lose Weight: An Astonishing Essential Oil Method"

"Turmeric: How to Use It For Your Wellness"

Therapeutic-grade essential oils are available from her company Sublime Naturals – be sure to use the discount code and link at the beginning of the book!

THANK YOU KINDLY IF YOU CAN SHARE A REVIEW OF THIS BOOK ON AMAZON!

Made in the USA
Middletown, DE
12 March 2019